Breathwork

A Simple Guide to Pranayama and Breathwork

(How a Daily Breathing Practice Can Drastically Improve Your Mind)

Caridad Cuellar

Published By **Tyson Maxwell**

Caridad Cuellar

Breathwork: A Simple Guide to Pranayama and Breathwork (How a Daily Breathing Practice Can Drastically Improve Your Mind)

ISBN   978-1-77485-788-5

No part of this guidebook shall be reproduced in any form without permission in writing from the publisher except in the case of brief quotations embodied in critical articles or reviews.

Legal & Disclaimer

The information contained in this ebook is not designed to replace or take the place of any form of medicine or professional medical advice. The information in this ebook has been provided for educational & entertainment purposes only.

The information contained in this book has been compiled from sources deemed reliable, and it is accurate to the best of the Author's knowledge; however, the Author cannot guarantee its accuracy and validity and cannot be held liable for any errors or omissions. Changes are periodically made to this book. You must consult your doctor or get professional medical advice before using any of the suggested remedies, techniques, or information in this book.

Upon using the information contained in this book, you agree to hold harmless the Author from and against any damages, costs, and expenses, including any legal fees potentially resulting from the application of any of the information provided by this guide. This disclaimer applies to any damages or injury caused by the use and application, whether directly or indirectly, of any advice or information presented, whether for breach of contract, tort, negligence, personal injury, criminal intent, or under any other cause of action.

You agree to accept all risks of using the information presented inside this book. You need to consult a professional medical practitioner in order to ensure you are both able and healthy enough to participate in this program.

TABLE OF CONTENTS

Conclusion

Introduction

In a variety of Eastern and Indigenous traditions breathing is considered to be an integral aspect of spirituality in the human experience. In this way of thinking, breathing could be confused with the spirit and frequently, the human lifespan is viewed in terms of the amount of breaths that are that have been taken.

When we think of breath is the process through which air flows into and out of lungs to aid in improving the oxygenation of the organs as well as eliminating carbon dioxide. This is the way that in modern Western societies we view breathingYi from a medical point of view. Breathing is a continuous process that is vital for cellular breathing and the elimination of carbon dioxide. It is mostly unconsciously controlled through the breathing center which is located in our brains.

We don't have to think about breathing , and generally, we do not. With our hectic daily lives it is common to see little connection between the breath we take and the various systems that are powered by it. The breath however is the essential fuel for our lives, and the manner in which we breathe has a profound impact on our mental and physical health.

With the constant pressure of tasks and stress of the day the automatic bodily function is rarely the first item on our mind. We seldom take time to think about breathing.

By using a handful of simple breathing exercises that can be integrated into our busy everyday routine, you can enhance our health, decrease anxiety and improve the energy levels of our bodies.

Chapter 1: Breathing Our Way To A Better

Life

The degree to how your breathing affects our overall health might not be apparent initially. This chapter we'll increase our knowledge of this complicated and often unthought of natural process by examining the various breathing processes (yes there's several!).

The benefits of breathing exercises will also be examined in depth using recent research that is based on evidence specifically in terms of depression and anxiety relief.

The Process(es) of Breathing

Although it is an unintentional and simple procedure, breathing involves a variety of and intricate interactions between the nervous system and the respiratory system.

How does our body learn to breathe? The breathing process is automatically controlled body function, similar to the heartbeat and digestion of food. The rhythm of breathing will be controlled by Medulla Oblongata the structure within the respiratory centre of the brain. It is a source of signals that control vital bodily functions. Alongside breathing rhythm, the respiratory system adapts the pattern of breathing to external or internal triggers.

The amount of breath cycles we take in one minute is a measure of our respiratory rate. The rate of breathing can vary in response to circumstances such as the impact of physical exertion or experiencing difficult emotional circumstances. It is possible to estimate your respiration rate by lying down by setting a timer to one minuteand then weighing your breaths. This method may not be 100% accuratehowever, since being aware that your breath is being recorded could alter your breathing patterns. Alternately, you can request someone else to take a deep breath, and then, as you rest in a quiet place, count your breaths for one duration of one minute.

The healthy rate of breathing is dependent on the life stage, and can vary between twelve and eighteen breaths per minute for adults (Eldridge 2013). A rate that is consistently different from the norm could indicate an underlying problem or an effect of certain behaviors like drinking alcohol or smoking.

The breath may traverse two distinct passages as it enters and leaves the body, namely the mouth and nose. In the ideal scenario, breath would predominantly traverse the nose because it's the ideal atmosphere for exhalation and inhalation. Nasal cavities are outfitted to allow air that is able to enter your body, such as by controlling the temperature of the air and moisturizing the air and cleaning dust, pollen and other contaminants.

Breathing is vital to draw oxygen in and also eliminate carbon dioxide. The oxygen we breathe is absorbed by the alveoli of our lungs before entering the circulation and carbon dioxide is released from our body via exhalation. Through our blood circulation, and specifically within the red blood cells of our body the oxygen inhaled is later transferred to the organs.

Thus, air quality is an additional element in this equation. Pollution from the air and poor the quality of indoor air are among the main causes of breathing issues and other health issues. Although, to a large degree, we can't manage the air quality around us, making sure that our homes are fresh, clean and free of chemicals can help in improving our health by improving the quality of our indoor air. To avoid the possibility of developing allergies to the air clean frequently and open the windows as often as is possible and keep clutter to a minimum.

Breathing is among the most fundamental ways we provide our systems with the components necessary to ensure they are running efficiently. After we've mastered the fundamentals of how we breath, let's look at the ways it affects our physical and mental health.

Mindful breathing can ease anxiety and Depression

As we've seen that the breath is automatically controlled to ensure our survival. It's not necessary for us to be reminded to breathe as our bodies are equipped with the right tools to ensure that our respiratory system is running well and adjusting to external and internal triggers. When we engage in physical exercise and our bodies require more oxygen, our breathing rate rises and the breath may become shallower. In the same way, when we're asleep or relaxed and sleeping, our respiratory rate slows down and the breath gets deeper.

It appears that this system is working effectively without intervention. Why would we need to learn breathwork?

The first thing to note is that our moods are closely linked to our breathing. There have been many instances of changes in the pattern of breathing due to changes in our mood. The connection between our emotions and our breathing is, however, in both ways. A deliberate alteration of the breathing patterns has been found to be a powerful method to alter the state of your emotions as well as in terms of improving mood as well as intensifying feelings of despair, insecurity and lonely (Philippot and co. 2010,). In one research participants were able to alter their moods by bringing particular emotions through imitating the breathing patterns that are common to either negative or positive feelings (Philippot and co. 2010,).

Recent research also shows that breathing with mindfulness can have significant effects on health particularly in reducing depression and anxiety. All of the methods described in this book are efficient methods to reduce anxiety levels, reducing stress and self-esteem, as well as increasing energy levels.

These are strategies that can help all through our lives to lead a more peaceful more relaxed, confident and also decide to employ in certain occasions in our lives when we require additional support. A study that was conducted with university students with extreme anxiety during tests found that the practice of mindful breathing daily helped significantly reduce the symptoms (Cho and colleagues. (2016)). The significant reduction in anxiety was observed in just eight short meditation sessions. In addition, the study pointed out that the positive results of the exercises affected how the students considered themselves and their internal dialog, even after they had completed the exercises. This suggests that breathing with mindfulness triggers positive thoughts that are automatic, even outside of within the framework of exercise which contributes to a more positive outlook on life.

Based on this research it is clear that breathing is a crucial technique to manage stress-related situations and to improve self-esteem. Its effects will last beyond the time spent in the exercise. It also proves that you don't have to be an expert in breathing to reap the benefits. Just a few sessions can be a significant step in improving your health.

In contrast breathing exercises may encourage healthier thinking pattern, as an study conducted by Jan M. Burg and Johannes Michalak determined. The study looked at ways that mindfulness breathing can help reduce depression and rumination for those who were unfamiliar with breathing techniques. Rumination refers to the negative repetition of thought patterns that cause negative emotions in a manner which increases the negative symptoms that are associated with these thoughts. It is a symptom that is common in various mental disorders, including depression and social anxiety, as well as obsessive-compulsive disorder and eating disorders as well as post-traumatic stress disorder.

This study was conducted over just one session, and it suggested an association positive between mindful breathing, alleviating depression and distancing from repetitive negative thoughts (Burg and Michalak (2011)). The ability to detach from ruminations, this study suggests, may have beneficial effects in the prevention of relapses to depressive episodes. As in prior studies the researchers found that mindfulness breathing enhanced the frequency of positive thoughts.

These findings point to the potential for breathwork. It is not just about decreasing depressive and anxiety symptoms however, it also has the potential to alter our thought patterns in general.

Instilling positive thinking will be the very first thing you do towards having a happier and healthier life. It can be done on it's own or in conjunction with other treatments breathing exercises can be the key to a more positive connection with ourselves and assist us achieve our highest potential.

Other health benefits associated with breathing work

The advantages mentioned previously aid in our general well-being and overall health. Mental and physical health are incredibly interconnected. A variety of mental disorders and illnesses can adversely affect our physical health and can cause physical symptoms.

However having a balanced mental state leads to higher energy levels, regular sleep cycles and eventually healthier bodies. In this way, any activity that has positive effects on our mental health will also benefit our physical well-being.

But the benefits of breathing work are more extensive. As we've seen, breathing is an essential function to ensure the health and health of the organs. The ability to provide adequate oxygenation to all cells in our bodies is essential for a proper reasoning as well as for enduring physical strain and healthy heart function.

Spending time breathing in a slow and deliberate manner will help in the proper function of the body's functions. This is through improving heart function and lowering heart rate, reducing blood pressure and relaxing muscles (Christophe Andre 2019). Additionally meditational breathing has been shown to be a significant relief from chronic pain, an observation which could transform the management of pain for those suffering from chronic pain (Zeidan and Vago 2016).

In this chapter, we've discovered the value of breathwork not just to enhance overall health, as well as to assist in managing specific health problems and challenges. Breathing techniques can assist the management of stress that you encounter daily and stress, as well as more serious issues or challenging life circumstances. Breathwork can be a great way to improve more of ourselves, all but without becoming an uncontrollable commitment that is difficult to reconcile with the other responsibilities we have.

Chapter 2: Breathing Through The Nose

This is where our breathing journey begins. The ability to breathe through the nasal passage is the very first stage to reconnecting with our minds and bodies, and in general, developing the habit of mindful breathing.

Mouth breathing that is frequent could indicate an underlying medical issue that can affect the quality of breath. We'll examine the various medical issues that can result in this respiratory disorder and also the environmental and behavioral factors which could hinder breathe through nose. Although in more serious cases of mouth breathing , a medical evaluation is recommended however, there are some practices and routines that can help facilitate breathing through the nose that anyone can benefit from.

Physical Characteristics that Hinder Nose Breathing

If you are constantly experiencing dry mouth and itching, halitosis (chronic unpleasant breath) or getting up exhausted or snoring or feeling exhausted all the time You could be taking too much breath through your mouth. Breathing is generally unconscious which is the reason it is possible that you don't even realize that you're doing it.

The act of randomly tuning into the breathing throughout the day and recording whether you breathe through the mouth or nose is a method to discover whether there is any issues in this regard. When you do this exercise, if you observe that you're breathing through your mouth, it's crucial to determine if you're feeling stressed or anxiety or any kind of exercise. If you can an easier way to conduct this exercise is asking someone else to observe your breathing and let you know if you're constantly breathing through your mouth.

There are a variety of ailments that can trigger breathing through the mouth which is why if you find you are breathing frequently through your mouth, especially when sitting, it's a good idea to consult medical professionals. Finding out if any of the underlying issues prevent your nose from breathing be the first step in attempting to resolve the issue and begin breathing more effectively for a healthier lifestyle. In any event, being knowledgeable of the major factors and signs that cause difficulty in breathing through the nose can be the first step towards looking for solutions.

Mouth breathing should be anticipated whenever nasal cavities are clogged. When the nasal congestion appears to be not permanent, for instance, it is caused by common colds, then the respiratory system is working exactly as it should and no further intervention would be required. If, however, you're having a lot of congestion because of recurring allergies, or sinus infections such as a sinus infection, it's worth it to seek a thorough medical exam to determine what is needed to ease breathing through the nose.

Another reason behind mouth breathing is the structure in the nose cavity. If the nose's structure, or even the jaw bone structure, makes breathing through the nose difficult air breathing in the mouth will occur more often (Cafasso 2017). A common instance is a deviated septum which can be corrected with surgery or other treatments. Other physical obstructions may be the cause of breathing difficulties including nasal polyps, growths of the skin inside the nasal cavity, and in some cases tumors (Cafasso 2017).

Sleep apnea is a further reason for mouth breathing, and requires special attention. According to Merriam Webster in the dictionary, sleep apnea is "apnea that is recurrent in sleep and is caused due to breathing obstruction or disturbance in the brain's respiratory centre" ("Sleep apnea," n.d.). Sleep apnea can cause breathing difficulties or shortness of breath breathing while asleep and is a reason to breathe by mouth. Since the body signalizes that it is deficient in oxygen and the respiratory system is triggered, it will try to fill in the gaps, and then go to the most efficient method to breathe.

It is also stated that, even after the obstruction is cleared there are some who will keep breathing through their mouths as a way of life (Cafasso 2017). This suggests the existence of a behavioural component to the problem and we can change our breathing patterns to healthier ones. There is no doubt that certain reasons for breathing through the mouth require medical intervention which cannot be substituted with behavioral changes. However, there is an element of behavior that is associated with mouth breath that could be addressed and improved with a few simple breath exercises that are mindful.

The Breathing of the Nose

After determining the medical cause of mouth breathing It is possible to increase the flow of air by the nose. Like most times when it comes to establishing and maintaining routines regularly, exercise is the most effective method to encourage breathe through the nose. Even if the majority times we're unaware of our breaths and exhalations and exhalations, we can train our body to subconsciously choose breath through the nose instead of mouth whenever it is possible.

There are many products available on the market to help with mouth breathing, including nasal strips, nose dilators jaw holders or mouth tapes. Based on the condition of the patient they can help ease breathing problems, however they do come with extra dangers. Internal nasal dilators could rupture inside the nasal cavity and create obstructions, and the use of mouth tapes can result in a lack of oxygenation while sleeping. An alternative that is more secure and safer alternative is to use saline irrigations. They are especially beneficial in cleaning and clearing the nasal passageway for sinus infections.

Additionally mouth breathing plays an important part in the body. In order to artificially block airway and force breath through the nose can cause imbalances within the system and miss the main reasons behind breathing problems via the nostrils. Our method is based on an encompassing view of our complex body, which recognizes and appreciates its intuition and wisdom.

Finding a way to tune with our breathing is the initial step of this process. Through this book, we'll discover the art of slowing down to honour the breath, respect the present moment and develop more healthy breathing patterns.

To accomplish this, we need to start by creating the right conditions that allow breathing through the nose to flourish. We must take regular breaks between work and other responsibilities in order to reset and reset and. A three-minute break every hour to relax the body, the mind and the eyes when you're working on screens, is bound to have a significant impact. By taking short breaks, you are signaling to your body and mind that they aren't required to work all day long, which lowers the stress levels.

A few minutes of short breaks to recharge and reset can provide an array of benefits to the mind and body in addition to reducing the chance of breathing shallowly. The majority of the methods we will discuss can easily be incorporated into three to five minutes of break You can also mix different elements of breathing to make sense during your breath journey.

In these brief and rejuvenating breaks, ensure you're not worried about the time being productive by cleaning up the house or re-reading tasks to be completed. It is more productive to rest and you can be sure that you're growing your mental capacity over the long term. Alternately, you can take a step up, particularly in the event that you spend a lot of time sitting in a in a seated position. You can lengthen your spine by raising the crown of your head as high as is possible, then lower the shoulders.

You can also encourage gentle and soft movements by performing some gentle stretching. If you are prone to the habit of being slouching in a slump or with a back that is hunched, you can combat this by interlacing your fingertips behind your back and pressing it down as you take 3 to 5 breaths with the nose, if you can. Depending on your back and shoulder flexibility, this could be a tense stretching of the shoulder, therefore be sure there's no discomfort or pain. An alternative to this exercise is to connect the thumbs, or keep your elbows bent.

If, in contrast you feel you have an aching spine it is possible to do a contra-exercise that will help relax. Begin by stretching the spine by standing up and moving your arms from left to right, and then all the way up. Take a couple of long , deliberate breaths as you extend your fingertips upwards towards the sky. Slowly move the fingertips all the way to the floor. It is possible to let your neck hang, and experience the deep elongation of the vertebras by vertebra. Be sure to breathe as deep as you can during these exercises, and especially when you are reaching down.

The short workouts, particularly when they are combined with breathing exercises, allow our bodies to ease up. Stress and fatigue are the most common reasons for the mouth breathing being shallow even though this might appear unrelated to the issue we're trying to address it is actually promoting breathing through the nose. Equally important is setting the time for conscious breathing exercises. The more we become aware of our breathing the more conscious it becomes and the more your body will learn to regulate it, making it more pronounced, slow and healthier.

Through this book, you will be taught breathing exercises that can be practiced during these brief breaks. This will allow the practice of unconscious breathing through your nose and prevent excessive breathing through the mouth. Breathing exercises that are specifically designed to relieve stress particularly can be a huge benefit to everyone, no matter the life style, or experience degree. In the next chapter , we will look at the typical mistakes that are keeping you from achieving your full potential in your breath.

Chapter 3: Common Mistakes: Bad Posture

And Mouth Breathing

It is believed that the breathing process, once seen self-regulated. Like the rhythmic motion of ocean waves the breath follows it's own rhythm. The exhalations follow the inhalations and so on without intervention from us. The way we breathe regulates ourselves in accordance with the requirement for greater or lesser oxygen to the body.

It might seem as if we're operating an engine that is well-oiled, so why should we make the effort to improve our breathing? Although it might appear, we're often breathing incorrectly. The internal factors we are unable to regulate can influence our breathing such as gender or age, weight as well as a myriad of health issues (i.e. chronic obstructive lung disease as well as chronic allergic reactions). There are various external and behavioral elements that affect our breathingpatterns, such as body posture, eating habits and the use of drugs, as well as the quality of our sleep. In addition external factors, like the quality of air, are a major factor.

Many factors that affect the respiratory system result directly from of our actions. After we have learned to begin breath through your nose we'll be able to look at what could do in our day-to-day lives that restricts the breathing. Making these mistakes can enable us to achieve the fullest potential possible and make the most of everything that breathing can offer us.

Breath and posture

Everyday activities put an annoyance to our posture. The rising trend of digitization in work is a good example. It shows that increasing numbers of workers spend at least eight hours a day sitting and frequently in poor posture.

Whatever the kind of workwe do it is commonplace to spend long hours in chairs that are not ergonomic in a crouching position, looking at our screens. "Text neck" is a relatively new phenomenon which describes the way in which constant staring at a smartphone affects the posture of the spine and posture as a whole. Back and neck pain is increasing commonplace ailments, and are which is a clear indication that the strength of the spine could be affected.

Exhalation and inhalation both work on our muscles in our upper bodies and organs. A poor posture could, consequently cause deep or compressed breathing. It is normal to breathe shallowly when our bodies are in stress or danger, and regularly breathing this manner signals our brains to be alert, which creates a'stress-like state (Ferris 2017). While shallow breathing is beneficial and useful in certain scenarios however, we require deep abdominal breathing to get the full benefits of healthy breathing.

Slouching constantly creates ideal conditions for a shallow breath because the posture can make it difficult to breathe in and exhale with ease. Inability to take deep diaphragmatic breaths, the necessity to replenish oxygen levels and rid carbon dioxide will force our bodies adjust to take more frequent breaths with your chest muscles. This could eventually cause a shortening of breath as well as fatigue and the escalating of the symptoms of stress.

Being in the same place for long periods of time and sitting for long periods of time does not support the optimal functioning of your body. The spine requires moving, so make sure that you take breaks from sitting for long periods and stretching regularly. This could be done in conjunction into breathing exercises that will be covered in this book. It will add benefits to your breathing practice.

If your workday is comprised of long hours spent at a desk You can begin with short breaks and stretching your spine. One method to achieve this is to spread your fingers, gradually lifting your hands upwards at the maximum height you're able to without elevating your shoulders, and then holding the position for 30 to 40 minutes. An alternative to this exercise, that gives your shoulders and spine more flexibility, is to join fingers or thumbs before lifting your arms up. If you are comfortable, you could then move your upper torso from left to right, all in one piece.

The spine, too, is not built to withstand intense physical strain that requires a lot of impacts, which is the reason running may cause damage upon the spine over time. If you're a frequent running enthusiast, it's advised to discover a balance and substitute certain workouts with exercises that help protect the spinal cord's integrity like swimming.

Our sleeping posture can affect the quality of breath. Sleeping positions that are not optimal can increase the risk that is sleep apnea. To ensure that you're breathing deeply during the night, do not sleep on your stomach to ensure that your spine is in a straight line. Instead, sleep on your side, and preferably with a pillow that is soft between your knees to maintain the alignment.

Emma Ferris, from the project in 2018 The Breath Effect, also recommends that we cut down on screen time to the extent feasible. Although this might seem extreme and inconvenient, when you consider the fact that the majority of our professional as well as social lives are online, it's feasible to achieve the right balance. Emma Ferris, health professional and public speaker, suggests we begin by creating the goal of having a day without technology that will undoubtedly bring many other benefits for our physical and mental health (2018).

According to this article, breathwork is a holistic method which considers the mind and body as a complete, intricate and interconnected system. Improved posture that allows for deep breaths is breathing, even if we're not doing any breathing exercises. In the next part we'll look at another method to help our breathing and general health by taking on one of the most frequent breathing mistakes: breath.

Do you think that mouth breathing is always bad?

As we've already mentioned the nasal cavities provide the ideal conditions for air to enter our respiratory system. The nasal cavities allow air for the lung by controlling the temperature of air as well as providing the needed humidity, and removing dirt and impurities (Emslie and others. 1952). The breathing through the nose also increases the creation of nitric oxide which enhances the absorption of oxygen into the lungs as well as oxygen circulation throughout the body. Furthermore breathe through nose can increase the resistance of the airstream, improving lung elasticity as well as oxygen retention (Cafasso 2017, 2017).

It doesn't mean, however that breathing through your mouth should be avoided in all circumstances. If air enters our bodies via the mouth and nose this is due to the fact that there are situations in our bodies that require both of the inhalation passages. The primary, and most obvious reason is that we have to breathe through our mouths whenever the nasal passages are clogged as a result of, say due to colds or allergy. Another scenario where it is required to breathe through the mouth could be when you are engaging physically strenuous activities that requires us to speedily replenish oxygen levels.

However, mouth breathing repeatedly is not the most healthy method to boost the oxygen levels in the mind and body, and could have serious health consequences. The negative consequences of frequent mouth breathing have been thoroughly investigated, including problems with development among children, specifically with regard to the facial structure, as well as damage to respiratory system's tissues caused by dry, cold and polluted air the increased risk of developing dental cavities and chronic fatigue (Emslie and others. 1952).

So, while mouth breathing is a physiological process and is necessary in certain situations for instance, when the nasal passages are overflowing, frequent breaths can be a sign of a more serious issue. It may cause health issues that span the entire body. Though it isn't often discussed it is a significant problem that could affect not only the quality of our breathing but also our overall health. In the following chapter, we'll go at this problem in greater detail and highlight some of the major reasons that may be hindering breath through our nose and also offering suggestions to help increase the amount of air that our noses breathe.

Chapter 4: Exercising Breathing To Help

Stress Relief

Many people think of breathing exercise as an method to manage difficult situations. Due to the speed of progress in the past few decades the pace of time is also increasing. Between work, daily chores obligations, and personal commitments it's easy to feel that there's no time left.

We are living in a fast-paced and productivity-motivated society. Our collective obsession with working hard leaves us with less time to enjoy ourselves and places less emphasis to reflection or rest. This is why it's not surprising that the majority of suffer from escalating stress, burnout, and anxiety-related disorders, like anxiety and insomnia are rising.

A few minutes every now or twice a each day, or at any time taking a few deliberate breathing exercises can create a all sorts of difference, and assist our ability to live a peaceful and more conscious life. These exercises will help you to settle the mind, pay attention to breathing, and enjoy the benefits of mindful breathing that will be carried over to all aspects of the day.

Belly Breathing

Diaphragmatic breathing, occurs as the belly expands every breath and shrinks upon exhalation, as opposed to breathing through the chest, which is less shallow. This allows for longer breathing, slowing, and relaxing breathing. The ideal scenario is that the majority of our breathing is belly breathing. Unfortunately, we're generally trained to compress the abdomen, which diminishes the chance of frequently breathing diaphragmatically.

Inhaling through the belly while wearing tight and tight clothes, or leading an extremely stressful life can all be considered as elements that can cause breathing through the chest. The practice of breathing in your belly is an excellent method to reduce stress and ease anxiety. The practice of belly breathing is also beneficial to our physical health since it can slow the heartbeat and may help to stabilize or lower blood pressure (Learning diaphragmatic breathingin 2016, 2016).

The breath of the belly is the base of all breathing exercises. Every subsequent exercise are based on the basic practices of this technique. It is possible to perform belly breathing exercises in a sitting position, standing up, down, or lying down. It is important to be relaxed and allow complete movement for the abdominal muscles.

If standing or sitting with straight backs is uncomfortable, you might be able to begin the exercise lying down, but preferably on an even surface or yoga mat. It is important to remember that straight back doesn't refer to a straight line from the neck to pelvis. The spine is naturally curvature that should be preserved. Instead of trying to imagine as a straight, geometric line, you should concentrate on lengthening your spine, and avoid the tendency to lean forward or backwards as you keep your shoulders in a relaxed position. For help in this exercise, imagine a string hanging from the top of your head. It will gently pulling you up and imagine that you are being held by someone as they gently pull them back down. Be aware of the elongation of spinal vertebrae and grounding your shoulders, as if were being gently pulled in two directions.

When you begin the workout, it is important to start with a few cycles of breathing naturally, preferring to do it by breathing through your nose. In the first breath cycle it is important to avoid forcing or controlling your breath. Posing in a relaxed position towards the breath could be an energizing practice on its own. In this state it is possible to scan your body to ensure you're not accidentally and inadvertently clenching muscles. This should be an opportunity to relax and releasing muscle clenching as an effective way to relieve tension and tension. Be sure to avoid tightening your jaw, face muscles, or your shoulders.

After at minimum three breath cycles, lift your left hand , and put it on your chest. You will then raise your right hand, and then put it on your stomach. This will make you more aware of where the air is moving as well as which muscle groups are stimulated. After that, take a deep breath through your nasal passage and sense the pressure of the air flowing downwards. Watch your belly rise and resist any desire to squeeze it. Place your hand gently on your belly. Watch the belly rising and falling, while trying keeping your hand and wrist in the exact spot.

While performing this exercise, you should not make any effort to inhale or exhalations. They naturally happen one after another So let your body manage the rhythmic sequence of exhalations and inhalations. Concentrate on the movement of your diaphragm. Feel warmness of your hands on your belly and feel the tension being released from your body with the exhalation.

If you're dealing with an anxious mind, you could practice counting your breaths on each exhalation This is a fantastic technique to help you focus your mind in the process of breathing throughout the day. Do at least 10 deep belly breathes throughout each practice, and allow your body to go through a few natural breaths prior to completing each exercise.

If you are relaxed and comfortable doing belly breathing lying down, you are able to begin to sit in a chair. The technique remains the same. The objective remains the non-observation of breath moving downwards when you inhale as the belly expands while softly contracting, and the hand moving with it.

The practice of sitting down can be a bit more difficult in the beginning because the posture may cause small abdominal compression that can lead to resistance to diaphragmatic breaths that are full. When you practice, ensure you're taking as much room as is possible, and keep your rear as straight as can. Standing straight isn't as simple as it seems as the back muscle needs to be strong. Do not get discouraged! By practicing, you'll increase the strength of your muscles in your back, and gradually sitting straight becomes easier. With more powerful back muscles, sitting becomes more natural and intuitive.

If you are able to comfortably perform at least 10 belly breaths from sitting You can also try to do breaths while standing. With your right hand resting placed on the stomach as well as the opposite hand placed on the chest, ensure that you're not leaning towards the front and that your shoulders aren't rising above your ears, or collapsing. It is important to create an elongated back and comfortable shoulders.

After you've practiced belly breathing through these three poses, you'll be able to begin slowing down each exhalation and inhalation until you've achieved an ebb and flow, organic, and rhythmic belly breathing routine.

This is an excellent exercise to tell your body to relax, reduce its pace, and be performed at any point and can be incorporated into a meditation routine. Apart from easing stress at a particular time it also contributes to an increase in unconscious belly breathing and nose breathing and better breathing patterns throughout the day.

Pursed-Lips Breathing

Have you ever felt that you were in such a state of anxiety that you could not breathe? In the majority of cases, when we are experiencing anxiety, we experience the sensation that our chest is swollen and we're unable to breathe enough air. When we experience panic attacks, we usually feel that we are not able to breathe deeply.

While experiencing intense sensations of panic attacks or anxiety cause it to appear that it's difficult to breathe most likely it is that we're not exhaling completely before initiating an additional breath cycle. In anxiety-related fight or response to flight, which are caused by the activation of our sympathetic nerve system the body is trying to absorb more oxygen than it normally. This is what will result in our system trying to breathe more frequently, however in a slower method. Inhalation is the only focus. could lead to the common sense that we're not breathing enough air.

The practice of breathing through the lips with pursed lips is an effective method to combat anxiety-related breathing shortness. The principle behind this method is that the exhalation can be controlled and extended. Contrary the belly breath, where our focus is predominantly shifted to the movements while inhaling, when using pursed lips breathing, we're going to focus more on exhalation.

Like the name suggests this breathing practice will require a change in the direction of the lips. The lips must be in a closed position during the exhale. It is possible to imagine placing your lips in a position like you're about exhale and blow away birthday candles or maybe to whistle.

It is best to practice the technique when sitting down, therefore it is best to be able to maintain a sitting posture prior to performing the breathing exercise with your pursed lips. You can also find an appropriate chair that can support your back, or lean against the wall.

Begin by getting into a comfortable and comfortable sitting position. To do this exercise you can lie on the floor, crossing your legs, in the chair or on the yoga mat. If you've been exercising those back muscles for a while, you could extend your legs front of you. This will give your entire body an extra stretch. This is an advanced posture since it requires more work from the muscles in the back to maintain the spine straight.

As you take a few slow breaths, try pay attention to your tongue. Then, to the best of your ability, separate it off the roof of your mouth. If you are at ease enough to begin the workout, start by inhaling air by breathing through your nose. After the inhalation, you'll purse your lips as you exhale slowly through your mouth.

The lips in the purse add resistance during exhalation however, it shouldn't be felt as if it is strained. If you feel the urge to breathe quickly after emptying your lungs you may have too much resistance. In this case, you may want to position your lips in an open "O" position so that more air can flow through.

Every time you exhale, bring focus to the rhythm of your breath. Take a moment to feel the air leave your body through your tongue, making a refreshing sensation on your tongue. Each time you exhale you will be able to visualize the anxiety disappearing from your body and your mind will be more peaceful and calm. If you're having difficulty in concentration or having trouble with racing thoughts This is a useful exercise because it provides new sensations and helps keep your mind in place while you are breathing.

Ten minutes of breathing throughout every session. It is an activity that can be done throughout the day, and for as many repetitions that you're comfortable with.

This approach will help your body naturally prevent the accumulation of carbon dioxide within your lungs. It can also help get rid of stale air, boost oxygenation, reduce the rate of breathing and reduce the levels of anxiety and stress (Nguyen Duong and Nguyen). It could also be beneficial for those suffering from specific health conditions, like chronic obstructive pulmonary disorder as well as panic attacks.

4-7-8 Breathing

This breathing method, commonly referred to as "the breathing pattern that relaxes" is a method created in the late Dr. Andrew Veil, aiming to create a relaxed breathing pattern that improves the oxygenation of our body. It also allows for the person to take control of the breath (Weil 2014). This breathing method has been demonstrated to be a potent anti-anxiety device and an effective approach to help you fall asleep (Gotter 2018).

In this practice we'll combine the lessons that we learned from the breath exercises and the pursed lips breathing exercises. We will also incorporate a count element into it. This is why it is crucial to practice these two exercises prior to attempting breathing in 4-7-8.

In order to begin for the first time, you should locate a comfortable seating place where you can remain still for a couple of minutes. Spend a few minutes to pay attention to your breath, stand a bit higher and loosen your shoulders. If you feel you are at ease and ready to start the workout and exhale with force all of the air remaining in your lungs by closing your mouth.

After the first exhale After that, move the tongue's tip to the rear of your front teeth on the upper side. The tongue should remain in this position throughout the entire duration of the exercise, creating some resistance while exhaling. To exhale more smoothly, move your lips to the position of a pursed lip, as previously in this exercise.

Then, take a deep diaphragmatic breathe through your nostril for the duration 4 times, then hold your breath until seven, then exhale in a slow, but forceful way through the mouth for eight.

The pace of counting will depend on your comfort level in the exercise and may be as fast or slow as you like. In lieu of being focused on the length of each count the Weil suggests that you focus on the duration of each count. Weil urges you to concentrate on keeping the ratio at 4-7-8 (Weil 2014). Typically being able to breathe comfortably can set the tone for the entire exercise. The breath you hold should feel at ease, not as if it is necessary to breathe in air. Find a pace that feels comfortable to you.

The doctor. Weil recommends starting the exercise with four breath cycles during each practice, and gradually progressing 8 breath cycle (Weil 2014). Eight is the number of breath cycles that are recommended for this specific exercise. After some practice, you will be able to gradually slow the workout, while making sure to maintain the ratio of 4-7.

This practice can help redirect the focus when you are experiencing anxiety and to manage cravings and to relax when you are experiencing anger or other extreme negative emotions. In this way it's an exercise that is suitable as a once-over to deal with specific emotions and situations. However The therapist Dr. Weil recommends consistent practice to get better results, particularly doing it twice per day. This can quickly boost the benefits of breathing for 4-7 breaths and create a peace and a positive outlook overall.

Chapter 5: Meditation Breathing To Help

With Depression And Anxiety

Meditation, which is the practice of mindfulness and distancing from thinking too much, is a process that is involved in breathing. Breathwork is often employed as a tool for meditation, to reduce thoughts and return the focus to the present. Regular meditation can help calm the mind, break free of the negative thoughts and increase confidence and self-esteem.

In this chapter, we will be taught how to combine breathing exercises and meditation specifically, to reduce depression and anxiety. We will do four breathing exercises designed to help you overcome overthinking, enhance self-love, experience deep relaxation and begin an attitude of gratitude. These exercises were created to make use of the foundations we've been working on to benefit from the practice of meditation.

How can meditation and breathing Incorporate?

Meditation is an ancient practice that dates back to the early Indian Vedas's writings the oldest written text of Hinduism. It refers to a higher state in consciousness, the practice of meditation is an integral component of spirituality across many religious traditions, including Hinduism, Buddhism, Islamism as well as Judaism.

The ability to block out distracting thoughts and concentrate your attention on something else was believed to be an indication of a higher level of consciousness, and the way to freedom. In the Hindu tradition the ability to master our minds will lead us to the state of divinity. The breath, according to the long-standing tradition was the vital force that led to the practice of meditation and gaining a firm grip on breathing patterns was an indication of rising.

Today, meditation has broadened its definition and techniques and is not restricted to only religions. Western societies may be a way to counterbalance their fast-paced and competitive nature and heightened competitiveness, have taken an interest in meditation and mindfulness. Although the methods we'll explore in this segment draw inspiration from the modern way of meditation, we remain steadfast for the spiritual and cultural roots of the ancient teachings.

The meditation exercises below honor the rich, ancient past and use the practice of meditation as a way to reach a higher level of consciousness. We hope these brief exercises will assist you in returning control over your thoughts, staying present in the present moment and developing a more positive connection to your self.

The practice of meditation is a great way to relax.

Many claim that they are unable to be able to meditate due to their mind running at a rapid pace and it's difficult to stop the continuous stream of thoughts that are erratic. This is precisely the kind of people who can benefit from a daily meditation routine.

Mindfulness is a process, not an ending point. There aren't any prerequisites required. You are able to bring your current condition of being into the practice, and it will be there for your practice in a total and unconditional way.

It can be a struggle to meditate. trying to slow down the speed of a mind that is racing can be like trying to stop a ball that is that is rolling down a hill. Once it begins to move. It is accelerating and eventually enough, it's out of control. Our minds are accustomed to being bombarded by an endless stream of information which reduces our attention span and hampers our ability to stay present. This is why whenever we try to slow down our thinking and focus on the present moment it could feel like the mind has a mind that is its own.

Because of this common issue in calming the mind, practices of meditation can trigger uncomfortable feelings of frustration, boredom and sometimes, negative thoughts about yourself. It is essential to relax and be at peace. The calmness that is evoked through a practice of meditation improves confidence and self-esteem and helps to reduce the feeling of being controlled by negative thoughts patterns.

The foundations we've laid down to date will ensure that you are equipped with the tools needed to conduct an exercise that makes you feel calm and rejuvenated instead of being disoriented and annoyed. The practice of focusing on breathing can be an effective method to control our thoughts and gain control of our thoughts. It can be used in a variety of ways however, it is particularly effective during meditation.

The next set of meditation exercises will incorporate mindfulness and breathing to maximize the benefits. The exercises will each be brief in order to be easily integrated into busy schedules, and it can be performed anytime, no matter what the time is comfortable. You can do each exercise in a sitting position, lying down, or standing up.

If you choose to exercise sitting down, you could be prone to getting sleepy during the workout. The possibility of falling asleep during meditation is normal and is healthy. It is a sign that your mind and body require rest, and you are able to return to the exercise at a later time. If, however, you're frequently sleeping in these exercises It is possible to shift to sitting for a couple of sessions.

There are a variety of soft ambient or soothing sounds, like ocean or water sounds to help you with the practice, or do these in silence, and pay attention to the sounds around you. Every meditation session will be different, based on the state of your mind and so you are able to revisit every exercise as many times as you'd like. Feel the various sensations that come up during every session.

Meditative Breathing to help with thoughts that are too frenzied and intrusive

If you find your mind spinning beyond your reach, and revolving around repetitive and circular thinking, then this program was specifically designed to help those who suffer from this. This meditation session will provide your mind with a needed break from reminiscing about the to-do list, reliving previous incidents, or worrying about the future.

Begin by slowly moving into the position you prefer which could be sitting with your legs crossed, lying on the floor with your arms extended gently by your side and standing. Pay attention to your breath, and feel your belly expand as you inhale and shrink when you exhale. If you are feeling comfortable you can close your eyes, or relax your gaze by looking a little downwards.

For the first few breaths take note of the sound and feelings surround you. Perhaps you can are hearing breeze outside the sound of children having fun, or perhaps the engine of a car passing by. Listen to the sounds around you, but don't label the sounds as pleasing or unpleasing.

You will eventually experience various thoughts surfacing and trying to divert your focus off of the present task. With no judgment and at the highest level of abilities be aware of what's happening within your head. Do not judge your thoughts let them all to be a part of your mind without hesitation.

Do not try to sway them away Instead, you should take note of the major aspects of the issues which are coming up. Are there any particular tasks that takes up all of your attention? Are you concerned about an upcoming event? Perhaps an interview or a job announcement? Are there any resentments due to be resolved? Do you have any difficult personal relationships? A past failure or embarrassment?

As you allow your thoughts to flow freely through your mind right now it is likely that you will begin to imagine the thought bubbles as that hover above your head. Each thought bubble is a representation of an unpleasant thought or emotion that you wish to release in these brief moments. Thought bubbles may be bigger, and some are smaller, it will depend on the amount of energy each one is calling for right now.

After taking inventory of every worry and thought, you are likely to be able to picture the thoughts descending over you. If you let these thoughts float within you, without dispersing them by force, you recognize their presence and significance. They are outside of you for the next few seconds, we'll be able allow ourselves to temporarily release them.

It is not necessary to discuss these issues right in this moment. You can simply signal to your brain that they're not in the past, and that you'll be back to them in the near future. This is time to dedicate to you. Be present in the present moment.

Slowly, bring your right hand up to your belly , allowing it to fully fill with air. You can feel your hand rising and then falling. You can breathe deep through your mouth or nose. You'll feel what is the best for you at the moment. If you feel it's right then exhale loudly through your mouth, making an sounds like 'SHH.

Each time you breathe you'll feel peace washing through your body. And with each exhale, you'll feel peace disappear from your body. The mind is in tranquility while letting go of all troubling feelings. Every breathing cycle, those thoughts that were hovering over you slowly begin to shift away, being pushed out by the air that is released when you exhale.

If you are confronted with a idea that keeps popping up You will be able to keep acknowledging it, and reminding you that it doesn't require attention right now. This is the time to sit with yourself. Whatever comes up is appropriate and is welcome. We are constantly returning to the breath as a method to ease away negative thoughts.

Pay attention to the way your body feels the moment. Take note of the relaxing effect that the exhale can have in your chest area, belly, and even your facial muscles. It is now possible to observe the thought bubbles moving farther and further away with each exhale like each exhalation creates the wind that blows them away. They're now far enough from each other that they've become blurry and nearly indistinguishable.

Relax for three to five breaths while counting them over your head in a whisper to yourself. Bring your focus back to your body sensations. Begin to feel the hand rise and fall on the rhythm of breathing. Slowly begin to make gentle movements with your fingers and toes. Inhale deeply through your nose and out through your mouth.

In the event that your eyes remain closed then open your eyes slowly while inhaling. When you are done with the exercise and moving on the next day you should take the time to be grateful for this time in a state of awareness. Your thoughts don't control you. You control your thoughts.

When you are well-rested, move your body and set yourself up to continue your day. This practice of meditative exhalation and visualization is designed to help you on your quest to have a more peaceful and more clear mind. It is possible to return to this practice whenever you notice your thoughts taking over.

Meditation Breathing to help Self-Love

Everybody has moments in where we are self-conscious, low self-esteem, a poor body image or feelings of being unworthy. This next breathing practice aims to bring out your best self and increase confidence and self-confidence. This is a quick routine that should be performed frequently to get the most benefit.

The exercise should be performed by sitting cross-legged or seated on your heels, knees and feet together facing the. If neither one of these positions is comfortable, place your back against an object or an appropriate chair that can support your back. You can also try standing up. For maximum benefit of this method it is recommended to stay standing up straight.

The first step is taking several deep breaths and confronting the doubt and self-doubt that could be rising up.

In the next exhalation deep You will look around your body to find the cause of the emotions. You might feel your chest tight, your forehead a bit heavy or your stomach to the point of knots or perhaps negative emotions stored in your hips.

In the following up to three or five minutes you will be focusing your attention exclusively on this region, and imagine the healing breath moving through the area affected. Each time you exhale, try to let the muscles relax even if it is a little. The body is slowly letting loose the tension as you breathe each cycle.

Next, shift your attention towards your spine. You will feel your back becoming more elongated, and your head standing high and confident. Inhale deeply through the nose and take a breath out of the nostril. Squeeze your shoulders a bit and feel the chest expand.

The next time you inhale switch your attention towards your belly. You can feel it expanding to make more space for the air coming into your body. Put one hand over the other , with your palms raised and move them slowly towards the belly. The core is a vital organ in our body and is a vital area for ensuring we are anchored and ensuring that our body is in a straight position.

Take note of any negative thoughts toward your belly are popping up, and then respond to them with a positive deep breath. If you're already acquainted to Ujjayi breath, also known as the breath of victory, you may start taking slow, full-depth Ujjayi breathing cycles. If not, be proud and enthusiastically take deep, deliberate exhales and inhale.

The next step is make your palms move towards the source of negative thoughts and feel the energy and warmth that is generated by the deep belly breaths there. You already have all the tools needed to get better.

As you deepen your breath, you could notice your hands' palms becoming warmer or energized by positive energies. Every breath triggers those hands' palms even more. Each exhale transfers the energy to the skin you're touching.

Being aware of the wisdom and divine nature that is your own body the radiant energy is spreading across your body, with its centre at the overlap of your palms. The next time you breathe in, Ujjayi or energetic belly breath, you'll be able to come up with something you feel proud of within yourself. If nothing comes to your thoughts immediately, you can take some more breaths.

When you've got it, gently whisper the mantra to yourself. Self-love can be a powerful and powerful tool. You are sufficient. You're doing your best. These affirmations will help you feel more self-love. The next time you inhale take a deep breath and feel the love enter your body. On you exhale, experience the self doubt disappearing from your body.

Your palms radiate warmth , which is radiating across your body. Keep your head up and lift your chin slightly and feel the self-love that is circulating within your. When you take your next breath you will feel as if the energy radiating through your palms is emitting an ethereal luminescence.

This light symbolizes the divine energy that exists inside you. It is all you require. Each time you breathe Feel this warm light get more and more powerful. You will now be able to see it's either orange, yellow or red. The warm color you see symbolizes your power within you.

The light is getting stronger and more intense. As it spreads throughout your body The glowing light will grow with every breath and will bring the divine energy into every part of you. You will feel your body is now immersed in warmth.

After a few triumphant breaths, repeat the earlier affirmations, either in your head or with a whisper. I am more than enough. Everything I require is in me. These are affirmations that you can go back to each when you feel a tingle of doubt in your own self.

If you're eager to return to your routine, gently bring your hands down. Do a deep, energizing breath, in and out to feel the positive energy flow throughout your body as well as your mind. Bring your hands up and relax across your entire upper body.

You're now ready to tackle whatever challenge that the day brings. Remember this state of mind whenever you're in doubt about your worth or position on the planet. You are sufficient.

Relaxation for the entire body

This breathing exercise will utilize the techniques of breathing to help promote relaxation and calm both in the mind and body. This activity can help reduce feelings of stress or anxiety attacks. It is also a good idea to practice it before bed to help prepare the body and mind to rest and combat insomnia.

In this workout it is a gradual relaxation of every muscle in order to attain complete relaxation. Thus, you must are able to spend at least 20 minutes of quiet time. The best way to do this is sitting down, so you should find the right yoga mat or towel to lay on. You could also lay on the bed if that is at ease. Before starting, shut off your cell phone and, to the best of your ability, get rid of any distractions in the vicinity.

While lying down, be sure you're in a comfortable position with your arms by your sides, and your legs extended and slightly wide. If you have your legs extended completely out in front of you for long periods of time could result in a sagging feeling in your lower back. In this situation you should lift your knees by gently placing a towel that has been rolled or a cushion under them.

The practice will begin with closing the eyes, and then turning our focus to the breath. Without trying to alter it, pay attention to the rate and quality of the breath. Spend some time observing the sensations that result due to the breath's movement upwards and downwards. Be aware of the temperature and quality of the air around you in the present.

When you practice this, try your best to let your breath flow effortlessly. As you relax, your breathing will become more deep and more sluggish.

If you are ready close your eyes and direct your attention on the inside. It is time to become an observer during the next few seconds. Take note of the position of your body and the relationship to your body and floor you are lying on. Consider what thoughts and emotions may be surfacing and allow them to pass through your mind.

The next time you exhale when you inhale again, you'll engage every muscle throughout your body. Engage your feet, your glutes, the leg muscles as well as the core, the shoulders, the arms and the facial muscles. On the next breath, ease your entire body onto the mat or floor. Experience the deep relaxation in contrast to the tightening.

Now is the time to begin the full-body massage. The next time you breathe in pay focus to your feet. When you exhale, let them release them to the fullest extent, making sure that you're not putting on any tension or grabbing your toes. Your attention should now shift to your feet. Make use of the soothing sound of exhaling through your mouth or nose to fully let your feet relax. They should be soft and then gently rotated towards the side.

Let's move through the leg and reach the muscles of the calf. Be aware of the relaxing effect each exhale brings to the muscles. If you feel the next breath come through your nose, turn your focus to your knees. Be aware of any discomfort or tension you may feel. When you exhale again relax any tension and release it you feel in your knees, feeling more heavy and the legs taking on a sinking sensation.

Feel the sensations now in your thighs. Relax those leg muscles relax more. Take in the comfort you are experiencing in your lower body. Breathe deeply and pay eyes towards your hips. Be aware of any tightness or pinching sensations, or any discomfort. The majority of us store our emotions on the hips. Without judgment, take note whether any unpleasant feelings appear. You're in good hands here. Let your body talk to you and take note of its messages.

The next time you exhale take a deep breath and let go of any tension you held in your hips. If you require multiple breath cycles to loosen your hips, it's acceptable too. You have taken this time to you. Pay attention to your body.

Begin slowly to ascend by paying attention to an area of your body that is inhaling, and then releasing tension when you exhale. Notice your belly rising with air and allow it to rise naturally and without intervention. Allow your body to feel weighty and sink deeper into the ground that you're lying on.

When you are at your chest, be sure to leave yourself as much space as you can by gentle pressing your shoulders back. Allow gravity to guide your shoulders back and down. Feel your chest expanding and relaxing. On exhale let it all go. Relax all muscles in your torso , and let your upper body relax however it naturally does.

After releasing your shoulders, lower into your arms till you are able to reach your hands. Be sure to move slowly and carefully. Keep moving in the rhythm of your breathing. Your body will determine the pace of this exercise. The expansion and contraction of your breathing to guide you through the next few minutes.

If your focus is on the fingers, observe the sensations that pop up. You might feel feeling of pulsation or tingling at your fingertips. Inhale and make a fist using both hands and then squeeze. When you exhale, let go of your tension, and you will feel the muscles relax. You can gently open your palms, signalling that you are open to whatever the universe has planned to you. You can also gently tilt the palms downwards and let your fingertips meet the surface. This is a sign that you're present and grounded in the present moment.

The body is sinking and deeper. Allow yourself to be completely present at this time. The calmness is slowly spreading over your body. When you are ready focus your attention on your neck muscle. If it feels comfortable then you can make some easy neck movements by tucking your neck a bit and lifting your chin. After that, find the most comfortable neck position and release.

Your attention should be directed towards your face. Relax your jaw If they're clenched or your jaw is tense. Relax your eyebrows.

Our facial muscles are usually stretched without even realizing it. Relax your lips parted and then when you exhale again take a moment to let your breath gently pass across your lips. Make use of this exhalation for a long time to relax all of your facial muscles.

Your entire body is at peace right now. For the next few minutes take a moment to sit completely still. Relax and let your breath be the sole movement within your body. Pay attention to the sensations. Feel the rising and falling of the belly caused by the air flowing in and out in a rhythmic manner, reminiscent of waves in the ocean.

When you're at ease and ready to begin your routine, begin making small movements with your toes and fingers. You can gently rub your index fingers and thumb with small circular movements. You can take a long, deliberate inhale through the nose. Then, after a long exhale, through the mouth, gradually let your eyes open.

Begin rolling your ankles and wrists to awaken your body. Moving your shoulders upwards, forwards, and back. Relax and take a few slow and gentle neck roll. Breathe through your nostrils while taking an entire body stretch.

Spread your arms over the top of your head. Spread your fingers and then firmly point your toes. The stretch should be held for a couple of breath cycles before releasing the stretch.

This method was created to bring deep relaxation for the body and the mind. If you're going about your day, move your body slowly to wake up and be able to take the peace that you gained to take with your. If you're ready to retire, lie down into a comfy position and relax to a peaceful and restful sleep.

Practicing Gratitude

This will be a quick practice that is easy to fit into your schedule and return to regularly as you require. You can do this meditation while sitting in a cross-legged position, kneeling with your feet resting on your heels and standing.

This will be a meditation that focuses on gratitude. Daily practice of gratitude will help to enhance your perspective on life and promote positive thinking. In this session we'll mix breathing exercises with affirmations for gratitude that give you a boost of energy and optimistic.

Begin by sitting straight and tall. Make sure you're not leaning to the side and don't let your shoulders slump. Begin by bringing your hands gently to your thighswith your the palms facing upwards or downwards or whatever feels more natural.

Consider someone you feel grateful to have this devotion. It could be a person you know, a family member or a colleague, or even your pet. Take a moment to close your eyes, or relax your gaze, and imagine whom you're doing this for. In your mind, say the affirmations below You are a blessing to me. your presence. Your presence makes my life more enjoyable. I wish you peace and happiness. peace.

Now, we will begin to work on our breathing. While you let the breath flow effortlessly, pay your focus to the breath. After two or three breath patterns, do an extended inhale with your nose and hold your breath for 2 seconds. After that, inhale through the mouth, making an "AHH sound as if you were fogging the windows of a building.

If you weren't able to catch it the first time around, don't fret We'll do it again. Inhale a fervent breath into your belly through the nose . Then, for a few seconds, take a deep breath. Inhale through your mouth while gently restricting your airflow like you were fogging the glass of a door or window.

We will utilize this breath's energetic power to awaken your feelings of gratitude. The next time you breathe in you, try to think of something you are thankful for. If you're having trouble to come up with something take a small step for this first time. When you've got it, hold the idea in your head while you hold your breath for a moment then exhale an exaggerated sigh from your mouth to express your gratitude.

We will repeat this exercise two times. Inhale and think of something else that you are thankful for. Remember it while breathing for a few seconds and then exhale loudly through your mouth. Consider a different thing you're grateful for today. Keep your breath in place, and then take a deep exhale with your mouth.

As you let your breath be restored to its normal rhythm, try to imagine your own image within your head. You can dedicate this practice to yourself by repeating in a quiet voice the affirmations below Thank you for your existence. Your presence makes my life more enjoyable. I wish you joy and peace.

Open your eyes slowly and be grateful for taking the time to practice gratitude.

Chapter 6: The Lessons Learned Of Yoga:

Pranayama Breathing Techniques

A lot of our current method draws inspiration from yoga's teachings on breathing, also known as Pranayama. In this section, we'll examine the key principles in Pranayama practice, and highlight the impact that yoga has left on breathing practice. We will also look at the evolution of breathwork using the perspective of yoga.

Then, we'll be taught four Pranayama exercises: Ujjayi, Dirga, Kapalbhati, and Simha breath. These breathing practices are more difficult than the methods previously taught. We will present a more progressive method that has a lot of variations to allow you to be patient and move at a pace that is comfortable for you. Through these four methods you'll gain a comprehensive understanding of the fundamentals that guide Pranayama practice.

It is the History of the Breath

Logically we can trace the history of breath back to the very beginning of time. For as long as there was life, there was breath. If we look for the first step of questioning the significance of breathing, individually as well as collectively, on the contrary, we're taken right back Hindi sacred texts that deal with spirituality, breathing and yoga as a single essential practice.

Yoga typically measures the quality of life by the number breaths that are taken, not how many birthdays that are celebrated. Based on this each person would be given the same amount of breaths during their lifetime. The ability to control your breathing and slowing the breathing cycle down could be able to, in the view of this theory enhance longevity. In the world of yoga breath is vital energy, connects the material world to the spiritual and acts as a vehicle for self-enlightenment.

Pranayama is a complex term in Sanskrit which is often translated as control of breath. The translation isn't but, in fact, accepted since every Sanskrit word can have a variety of meanings. To clarify the meaning of what the term means, Kathy Phillips (2002) provides the following explanation:

Prana can mean a variety of things in Sanskrit. It's not just the word that means breathbut life force cosmic energy, air and force as if yoga could not differentiate between breaths of an person and the energy of the cosmic. (p. 123)

In spite of our current understanding of yoga as a sequence of postures that improve the flexibility and strength, in the beginning yoga was primarily focused on breathing exercises and meditation. Indeed, the narratives in the Rig Veda texts, believed to date around 1000 B.C. between 1500 and 1000 B.C., significantly emphasized the importance of breathing exercises and meditation over asana that is the sequence of various postures for the body (Singh 2021).

In the Vedic period breathing exercises were performed as part of an a cultural and religious context. One of the primary goals was to improve lung capacity so that it could enable continuous singing of mantras during prayers (Singh 2021). Knowing how to hold breath was also an important aspect of religious ceremonies. In this period the breath was linked to attaining spiritual height, via breath, and also with grounding in the physical world through exhalation. Additionally in the event of being in a position to hold breathing, one can be able to master the body through the mind.

It was not until the Patanjali period that Pranayama was first recognized as a part of religions. It was only during the Patanjali period that Yoga Sutras of Patanjali (early descriptions of the yogic principles) defined Pranayama as being one of eight yoga limbs that included asana, physical exercise of meditation, moral discipline and enlightenment among others.

Due to the increasing popularization and popularity Hatha yoga, particularly after the 16th century, the practices of yoga have been putting increasing importance on physical postures and the improvement of one's self by moving the body. Following an initial Hatha Yoga revolution in the sixteenth century, scales tilted slightly , and physical practices began to take on the breathing, and eventually became a complement to the earlier.

Today, we typically think of breathing as a way to attain other purposes. We might practice deep breathing to strengthen our minds, or we could learn to manage the breath to increase endurance during workouts. In the first interpretation it was opposite. The asanas, also known as yoga postures were viewed as tools that could be used to concentrate the mind and learn to master breathing. The actual work was taking place within the mind in the body, and via breath.

Even though Pranayama nowadays occupies a lesser place in yoga practice, particularly when we consider Western modern yoga interpretations the teachings of this ancient tradition still have significance even today. The methods we'll be learning next, supported by more anatomy knowledge, are derived from ancient teachings that help improve clarity of thought and concentration, self-esteem and energy.

Pranayama Breath

In the next part we will review the four major breathing techniques that stem from the ancient yogic practices. They will be an increase in difficulty from the breathwork exercises that we have covered in the past. Take breaks whenever you need to and try every step several times before proceeding to another step.

Each exercise will be presented in distinct stages, and they will be introduced in a gradual manner. The difficulty of exercises will gradually increase. We suggest that you do each exercise as long as is comfortable for you and gradually progress through the exercises. Although you might want to master quickly and completely every workout, those are exercises which take time. Therefore, it is suggested to take an approach that is gradual.

Nadi Shodhana Alternate Nostril Breathing

Nadi Shodhana breath is commonly called"the alternate nostril breath is a common practice in modern yogic circles. This is explained by the relative ease of this method, and also its numerous benefits. Because it requires breathing and coordination of movements this is a fantastic exercise to improve focus or to soothe a stressed mind.

Because breathing through the alternate nostrils is a partial obstruction of nasal cavities, this may not be the right choice when you're feeling sluggish. In addition it can be used by anyone, anyplace, and any time.

To learn to the alternate nostril breath, start by finding a comfy sitting down posture. Find your balance, ensuring the spine of your straight while your shoulders remain slack in the back.

In the beginning to begin, take three breaths through the nose , and then out again through the nose. Through this exercise, air will only circulate through the nose. It's beneficial for those who want to breathe through your nose more often.

When you're ready to begin your exercise, raise the hands of the right and then lower your middle finger and index finger, while keeping the thumb and rings fingers extended. It is also possible to soften the little finger , or extend it, but it is more comfortable. Depending on the flexibility of your hand the position you hold for an extended period of time can be uncomfortable. Alternately, you could alternate nostril breathing using your thumb and index fingers extended.

To begin, place your thumb towards your right nostril and stop any air flow. Take a slow inhale through the left nostril while your right nostril is shielded with your thumb. After you have inhaled, holding the thumb in place grab the ring finger and wrap your left nostril. Then , let the air out by opening the nostril on the right with your hand lifted while making sure that the ring finger remains in the correct position.

Now, we will duplicate the exercise in a mirror mode, mirroring your movements your hand on the left. Make sure that the ring finger is over your left nostril in order to allow you to breathe through your right nostril. When you are at the top of your breath take a moment to cover your right nostril with your thumb and keep the breath in for a few seconds. Release the ring finger and exhale through your left nostril.

If you hold your breath, ensure that you don't feel any discomfort, or do not feel the urge to breathe immediately after the breath. Breathing in only one nostril could cause tension in the intake of air particularly when we are being a bit congested. So ensure that you're not experiencing the desire to breathe more quickly.

If breathing is uncomfortable, it is possible to begin working on the exercise without the hold first, and afterward add it until we feel at ease with the exercise. The practice without holding the breath reduces the complexity of the exercises making it much simpler for those who are new to the sport.

For a simplified version you can also begin with some deep breaths in both nostrils prior to putting your hands in a position using either the fingers extended, the thumb and ring finger or by extending the index and thumb to make it easier. When you're ready, move the thumb towards the right nostril while inhaling by breathing through your left nostril. After that, move the ring or index finger towards the left nostril, allowing the air to pass into the left nostril. Keep the ring finger in the position of inhaling into the left nostril. Then immediately cover the right nostril with your thumb to exhale out of the left nostril.

Continue to practice these sequences until it becomes more natural. Do at minimum six breath cycles per session. This method requires coordination and practice. Keep the rhythm steady and changing the nostrils after each exhale. Be sure that at the conclusion, you've taken an the same amount of breaths, ensuring you've breathed and exhaled the same number of times through each nostril.

If you feel that you are in a good position on alternate nostril breathing you can work on extending each phase of the exercise , and gradually becoming more comfortable in breathing between the inhale and exhale.

If you are patient and consistent the technique will keep your mind alert and focused by connecting the brain with the body. If you believe you've mastered this method practice, breathing with alternate nostrils is a powerful method to combat anxious feelings, or even to help you pull yourself away from panic attacks.

Dirgha Three-Part Breath

It is the practice that Dirgha (also known as three-part breath) is a way to take the principles of belly breathing and extends the range of these lessons. The practice helps to increase awareness of the path that the air takes through a breath. This breathing method creates the deepest breathing possible and also has profoundly calming effects which is why it works well with meditation that is deeply relaxing. Through incorporating both diaphragmatic as well as breathing in the chest, three-part breath gives the most oxygenated oxygen to cells, enhances lung capacity by allowing them to reach their maximum capacity and also increases the strength of the abdominal and diaphragm muscles (Bilski 2019).

For people who are just beginning, this exercise should be done lying down. Once you feel more comfortable then you can shift the exercise to a sitting posture.

The first step of this Pranayama exercise is practicing comfortably belly breathing. If you're not fully confident in your abdominal breathing it is possible to go back and go through our instructional guideline for this fundamental breath until it is natural. The practice will start by taking five slow and deeply diaphragmatic breathings.

Breathing in the belly is something that should be natural however it isn't always. To assist your breath move down into the diaphragm area, place the right hand on your lower belly. Focus your focus on the path that the air travels until it fills the belly by raising your hand. Begin by taking five slow , deep belly breaths.

While keeping your right arm on belly area, bring the left hand toward your ribs. When you inhale the next time you will feel your belly rising by air, and then increase the inhale until it reaches the rib cage region. The right hand lifting, and then the left hand rising just a little. The lungs are now filled with a little more air than you would with simply breathing in your belly. When you exhale, feel the rib cage expand and empty. Then, you can feel your belly contract and empty, as slowly that you are able to. Do five more breaths similar to this one.

Let the breath be as relaxed as you can. The goal is to control the direction of your breath through your mind and not forcing your muscles to contract or expand.

After at least five minutes After five breaths, move your left hand into mid-section of the chest. The next step is to let the air expand to the chest. Inhaling the breath, slowly let the belly fill up with air, followed by the chest, then the rib cage. the chest. When exhaling, be sure to go in the opposite direction. In the beginning, you'll clear the chest before moving to the ribcage and then your belly.

Keep practicing for at minimum five breath cycles.

If the breath is moving through the ribs to your chest area, it is helpful to lower the chin a bit so that there is more room for the air to take up. If you're struggling to discern between distinct zones, this awareness will develop through time and repetition. We're not taught to focus on our breathing and, as a result it's not a surprise that there could be an inconsistency with the internal processes involved in breathing.

Doing the three-part breathing will increase the awareness of this, slow the breathing, and place you in the present and in the present moment sensations. It is also an effective tool for relaxation exercises that are full of body or when getting ready to go to sleep.

Ujjayi: Victorious Breath

Ujjayi Pranayama that means victorious breath, is among the most fundamental practices in Pranayama practice. Yoga sequences of all kinds are fuelled by this breath of victory, particularly because of its calming and energizing effects. The slight constriction of the throat's back as well as the sound that air creates when it passes through, helps to settle the mind, fill your body's energy and establish the pace of the yoga movements. Also known as ocean breath Ujjayi Pranayama is easily recognizable due to its distinctive sound, which sounds like waves breaking against the shore.

The breath technique releases energy, strength and provides a groundedness. It is therefore best to practice it while standing or sitting. Find a comfortable spot to stand or sit for a couple of minutes and find an area to lengthen your spine, and then ground your body.

Begin by focusing your attention to your breath, and make sure you're inhaling and exhaling through your nose. Ujjayi breathing can be described as a method that is solely based on the breath of the nose. Therefore, make sure that you're at ease breathing only through your nasal passages for the next couple of minutes before you begin.

Take a long, deliberate inhale with your nose, and upon exhaling, you can make sure to exert some pressure on the air passage by contracting the muscles at the back of your throat. Inhale for five breaths after which you attempt to exhale loudly, but without opening your mouth.

If you're struggling to create the distinctive Ocean breath sounds, first be aware of the actions which must take place within the muscles of your throat in order to create the small restriction. After another long inhale with the nose, exhale through the mouth loudly like you're inhaling a glass of sludge.

You can also take your hands, put it over your mouth then feel warm exhaling through your mouth. Try this for two breath cycles. After the third exhalation try closing your mouth when exhaling. Make efforts to maintain the same air-restriction you experienced before. In the following breath cycles, you should begin exhaling by breathing out while keeping your mouth open and closing your mouth halfway through exhalation.

As you close your mouth, pay attention to the back of your throat to ensure that you maintain the soft restriction of your airway. If you're in need of more practice then take as many breaths of practice as you can. After closing your mouth in during the breath, observe whether you hear the gentle sound of air passing. It is not intended to be loud or a stricture and so, seek out an inner whispering sound.

If you are able to maintain this restriction when closing the mouth The following step will be to maintain your mouth shut and breathe through your nose throughout the entire practice. In the following breaths, take a deep breath, and feel the slight constriction in the back of your throat as you exhale. Feel the grounding and revitalizing impact of the sound of the ocean radiating throughout your body.

After you feel you've are in control of the constriction in the exhale, you begin the full Ujjayi breath practice. Keep the constriction for the entire length of the breath. Finding the sound of the ocean may be a bit more difficult during the inhale. Set your attention by focusing on your breath, as you feel air rubbing against the back of your throat in order to bring you back into the present.

Continue to practice until it becomes naturally. It is then possible to use this breath whenever you need a boost of energy or a way to anchor your scattered or busy mind. When this breath sounds more naturally, and without needing to pay attention to the mechanics of it, Ujjayi Pranayama works particularly when you are moving.

As previously mentioned asana yoga exercises are often a guide to focus on Ujjayi breath to establish the time frame at which you change between poses. Since this is an energetic breath, it is also able to be activated in more intense physical activities, like running. Ujjayi breathing stops hyperventilation, and encourages an even and consistent air flow coming into as well as out.

This function of regulation along with the power of anchoring the sound of a soft breath, makes this technique a great method to combat anxiety, and also to help us return to our present situation when we are experiencing the time of a panic attack. In the end, it is a breath technique that is versatile that, though it can be difficult to master initially, it more than compensates for it with the benefits it offers.

Simha"Lion's Breath"

If you're overloaded with negative energy and are in need of to release tension, the Simha Pranayama is the perfect breathing practice to let go of tension. Just press on the button to refresh. The forceful exhale from the mouth will release any negative feelings leaving you feeling strong revitalized and brimming with confidence in yourself.

The breathing technique is simple to master, however the challenge with this Pranayama exercise is in maintaining the lion's breath posture. So, prior to putting the entire exercise together, we'll focus on understanding the breathing techniques of Simha Pranayama.

Let's begin by getting to a comfortable position. If sitting on your heels is easy, then you can begin by preparing to advance the practice to an entire Simhasana, also known as lion's posture. If you want to take it one more advanced step, you can start by lifting your heels off the floor and keep your toes curled under you and seated on your heels. This is a very deep stretchthat may become extremely uncomfortable after a few minutes. To improve flexibility in your feet, you could alternate lifting your heels while keeping them on the floor.

If you are experiencing knee pain or knee pain don't push yourself too hard. It is possible to do lion's breath exercises sitting comfortably or even on a chair.

Begin by gently pressing your hands towards your knees and permitting your chest to relax and relax. As you watch the breath flow through and out of your body, focus on the area just over the middle of the eyebrows and right above the nose. This is referred to in the yoga practice as the third eye.

Based on the first concept of the Third Eye it is a powerful intuitive center, which is a gateway into a higher level of consciousness that is watching over us and ensuring that we are in the right direction. Physically it is believed that gentle pressure on the third eye can create an uplifting effect. You can experience the relaxation potential in the eye's third by gently massage it using your fingertips in an upward motion.

With the intention of focusing on the location and the existence in the 3rd eye. take a deep breath through your nose. When you exhale take your mouth open and let out an exaggerated "AH" sound. Sigh. Breathe in again through the nostrils and then exhale. take the same forceful and loud breath out , however this time, you should extend your tongue as far as you can during the exhale. Inhale a second time through the nose, then at the exhale, look upwards and down as if you were looking directly into your third eye.

This practice may appear to appear silly at first. Use this time to let off any shame or discomfort and completely engage in the exercise. You might feel that you're tempted to be a joke about the situation or yourself and that is acceptable. Breathwork doesn't have to be solemn or serious. The breath of a lion is a wonderful way to inject some levity into breathing exercises.

After we've learned about the various aspects of lion's breathYi , looking to the eyes of the third breathing out in a loud voice through the mouth and exhaling the tongue outYi, it's time to put all of them together into one big breath. Breathe in through the nostrils and then on the exhale, look up and into the air, then allow a loud breath out of your mouth. Then, extend your tongue towards the cheeks.

After some practice, you'll be able to gradually increase to 1 lion's breaths. At the moment you can take as many lion's breaths as feel comfortable. Let all negative energy go after every exhale.

If you are comfortable with going a step further, then we can begin to work on Simhasana which is the full breath of a lion. This is a tense posture that requires an intense stretch of your body as well as flexibility. Be patient and don't overstretch and pay attention for your body.

Begin by stepping onto the floor or to a yoga mat, and then sitting on your heels, keeping the legs firmly together. If you feel this is already an extreme stretching, continue doing this exercise in small increments prior to going to the next stage.

To push further To go further, place your glutes on the heels while flexing your knees to the left and right. Take your hands slightly inwards and place your palms in the flooring. Be sure to avoid lifting your hips, or overarching your lower back. The goal is to maintain the lower back solid while maintaining the stability and stability of our spine. You'll feel a firm stretch in the hips, along the sides of the body, and on the upper thighs.

When you're allying breathwork to posture, be sure that your posture does not restrict your breath in an order that isn't able to allow complete abdominal breathing. If you're having trouble trying to fill your belly up with air, step back and then practice the previous technique for longer until you feel at ease to advance. The next point of reference is to curl your toes and raise the heels while remaining in a lowered hip. This will increase the depth of stretch, and will put your feet' flexibility up to the challenge.

The final step in achieving Simhasana in its fullest form is to turn your hands inwards and stretch the arms. Take the right hand up and rotate your hands completely to the left so they face towards you. If they don't go completely it's possible to keep them at a half-way point, with your fingers pointing towards the right. Slowly and slowly place your hand on the floor or on a yoga mat. After that, lift the left hand and turn it completely to the left, so that your fingertips are facing your lower body or as much as it can comfortably turn before putting it back on the mat or floor. It is possible to practice this by turning and putting each hand one at a moment until you are able to hold each hand in a place for a few seconds.

After you've completed this exercise and have stretched your wrists, arms and hands sufficiently to the point that you want to turn both hands towards you in an entire lion posture. If you're in the position be sure to take a moment to appreciate the strength of this pose. Keep your shoulders and arms engaged so in order to avoid collapsing into your wrists. Once you're ready, take a deep breath through your nose, then let the breath flow out on the exhale using a full lion's breathing posture. You can do as many as ten lion's breaths during your practice, stopping when you experience any tension or dizziness.

Feel this fresh, deep energy flowing throughout your body, moving across the third eye up to your throat, along the spine and onto your muscles. Keep your mind and body active, and make use of the forceful exhalations you can make to let go of everything that doesn't serve you.

If you practice it with care breathing and lion's posture are excellent tools to transform negative energy into positive self-loving, optimistic and optimistic energy. Whatever level of practice you're in it is the energy boost you require after a long and difficult day. The ability to let off unnecessary feelings is essential to living an easier, more relaxed life. And lion's Breath can help you achieve the direction you want to go.

Kapalbhati Breath of Fire

The final Pranayama method we'll be studying will be one called the Kapalbhati breath, which is commonly referred to for its breath of flame or the breath of skull luster. By its short and swift breaths, Kapalbhati purifies the airways and strengthens the body and removes the toxins. It is a breathing exercise with regards to difficulty therefore, before you begin the practice, make sure that you've done other breathing techniques and are already feeling a connection with your breath.

Breath of Fire is purifying energetic, invigorating, and cleansing breath that helps to get you moving and prepares your mind and body for moving. This is why this Pranayama exercise should be practiced in the morning or in the early afternoon. Additionally, this method relies on controlled hyperventilation which is why it should not be performed if you suffer from hypertension or any heart-related complication or vertigo. This method is not recommended for those who are expecting.

After ensuring it's safe to practice Kapalbhati Begin with sitting. If you are more comfortable with the method, Kapalbhati can also be performed sitting on the floor. For now you should begin by sitting up straight and tall and sifting throughout your body to check for clenching and tension that is not needed.

It is an active breathing. This means that we'll press it rather than watching it. This is why it is normal that our bodies tighten up and contract during the initial exercises. Pay attention to the facial muscles and make sure your jaw is relaxed and that the muscles of the eyebrows are not strained, and that the forehead is at ease. If you require further adjustments to your posture then feel free to do your time during this exercise for example, rolling the shoulders upwards, forwards as well as backwards, and doing several slow neck roll.

Kapalbhati utilizes breathing through the nose passively and quick forced exhalations via the nose. Bring your right hand towards the lower belly, and hold it there for the duration of the practice. In the beginning, take some time to watch the breath cycle for a couple of breaths and note the quality of your breathing. Take a breath more and expel the air from the nose, by firmly contraction of the diaphragm.

Inhale deeply, then take another slow and quiet breath cycle. Then, after the next inhalation take a deep contraction of the muscles in the core and then expel the air from the nose. Repeat the exercise one more time, allowing one passive exhale and inhale and when you sense the next inhale getting stronger, you should be exhaling air by contracting the diaphragm. After the third exhale, which is a forceful one then put your hands down and relax for a minute.

This method stimulates the deep core muscles. It is normal to notice some energy or perhaps soreness in the core. Through practice, Kapalbhati is also a fantastic way to build the strength of your core in addition to improving posture. Begin to build up the practice slowly by noticing the different effects on your body.

If you are you are ready to go deeper in your practice, we'll to speed up and shorten the exhalations. Be sure to ensure that the inhalations are gentle and passive. We only desire to make the exhalation more forceful. Reposition the hand back to the belly area and begin to observe the breath cycle for a few breaths. Once you are good enough, you can begin contracting your diaphragm quickly, speeding the beat for as long as you feel as comfortable. In the beginning, for the first few rounds, you should not overdo it with ten sharp exhales. And make sure to allow a few full breath cycles between rounds.

Pay attention to any indications of overheating or dizziness, you can increase the intensity of your exercise by extending the time spent in the exercise , and intensifying the pace of your abrupt exhalations. As the speed increases you will begin controlling both the inhalation as well as the exhalation. But, make sure you're keeping your inhale relaxed and your abdomen soft as the air is entering.

The perfect way to get us awake from a deep sleep, Kapalbhati should not be performed regularly or for prolonged durations without interruption. Keep the breath of fire to use at times that you need an extra boost and let the benefits of this energetic full-body experience spill over into your daily routine.

Chapter 7: Breathing When Training

Our breathing cycles are created to help us stay in our position while we move. This is why our respiratory rate changes according to the intensity of physical activity and consequent requirement for oxygenation. When you are engaged in vigorous physical activities there is typically a subconscious reflex to begin taking deep breaths, or to even keep the breath. When exercising for a long time it could appear as if it's impossible to take deep breaths. In this article we will dissect and examine the connection with breathing, and activity.

In addition, while it's not the main focus of exercise plans, correct breathing during exercise can improve efficiency and result in the success of your exercise. This article will provide most effective breathing techniques to use when exercising to maximize the benefits of your exercise routine.

You may be holding your Breath During Exercise

Have you ever been in an inverted plank and realized you held your breath all the duration? Have you ever struggled to coordinate your breath and movement during exercise?

This isn't surprising, due to the disconnect between breathing and movement. When we learn new exercises, it's not often that we are taught to breathe during the exercises. Fitness instructors can remind us at times to breathe in but it's equally important to be aware of what to do and when to breathe.

We have all the tools to identify the correct breathing pattern for various types of exercise. Rule one is to always pay attention to your body, and listen to the needs of your body.. Focusing solely on the outcomes, constantly challenging our bodies to its limits, while ignoring the quality of our breath while doing exercise can make for an unbalanced and ultimately, harmful method of working out.

Breathwork techniques like the belly breath, Ujjayi breath, and the pursed-lips breathing are incredibly flexible to various types of exercise. In the following section, we'll dive into the most effective breathing techniques to ensure you're getting all the benefits of working out.

The proper way to take your breathing while exercising can improve endurance and flexibility. In contrast the act of holding your breath can cause stiffness, which can lead to a decline in endurance, and could cause fainting or dizziness periods. It is essential to replenish the oxygen levels in our body, particularly when we're straining the muscles and pushing ourselves to the limit.

Breathing through the Moves

Exercise can release endorphins and improve our mood that improve our mood, sleep patterns, and increasing our energy levels. Furthermore, if it is done mindfully exercising regularly, it increases your breathing capacity and provides therapeutic benefits to those suffering from asthma or other breathing issues. But, as we've seen when we're consistently keeping our breath while breathing, or breathing slowly or hyperventilating, then the negatives could outweigh the advantages.

A well-planned exercise routine should be based on appropriate breathing techniques as a fundamental element of the exercise. This can greatly improve the effectiveness of the exercises and also to the long-term viability of the exercise routine.

In general it is important to keep our breath in a steady rhythm when exercising. It is possible to achieve this by synchronizing movement and breath. If, for instance, you're running take each step as a chance to determine the pace of breathing. Inhale for three steps then exhaling for four steps. Allow your breath to establish the pace of your practice, and then adjust when necessary. If you feel your breath becoming less pronounced, listen to your body's signals that you may have to slow down.

It is also possible to synchronize your breathing with other kinds of moves. If you're doing weight training, completing all breathing cycles is essential because it can prevent hernias and can signal if you're carrying too much weight. If you can't breathe throughout an exercise, you're exaggerating your body and should consider taking the step back. When lifting weights, take a deep breath through your nose in order to return to your original position, then exhale through the mouth or the nose to tighten and raise. This ensures that even during the most strenuous movement we are fueling our muscles with oxygen.

However core exercises can present some challenges that are a bit more challenging. As we all know, the muscles of the core are crucial for the inhalations and exhalations as they provide the motion for air to flow inwards and outward. If you are doing sit-ups or crunches Inhale slowly through your abdomen, and then on the exhale, contract and raise your upper body. This way, you're still breathing in fully and strengthening your muscles in your core.

If the primary exercise is based on keeping the core muscles contract as in the plank, you may appear impossible to hold deep belly breaths like there is no room, or as that it could seriously weaken the posture. To combat this it is possible to follow the principles of three-part breath and let the breath reach the rib cage. As you exhale you should try to relax only your lower belly, leaving a little room in your rib cage. When you inhale again will feel like there's more room for air to enter.

Make sure to continue to take breaths through your nose. It is possible to think that exhaling through your mouth is required to let heat out and expel the air faster.

In the end, you'll find that any among the techniques for breathing that we discussed can be beneficial while working out. Breathing in the belly should be done throughout the day and is suitable for most exercises. Ujjayi breath is a good option in more intense workouts because it assists in setting the pace for movements and provides a sound to hold the attention in place and helps to oxygenate the body in a way that is efficient. Pursed-lips breath can also be used for intense workouts since it permits a complete exhalation that reduces body temperature and helps replenish the lungs with fresh air.

As we are able to see, the power of breathing can be seen in every aspect of our lives. We can take its lessons to us and implement them to all areas of our lives, allowing us to witness the positive benefits that mindful breathing can bring to our mental, physical, and spiritual health.

Chapter 8: Modern Holistic Approaches:

Soma Breath And The Wim Hof Method

The breathing practices we've discovered so far adhere to traditional teachings from the past, and continue traditions that were for centuries utilized in religious circles and are only now entering mainstream circles. As we've discovered that mindfulness is not exclusively practiced in religious circles and has expanded to a variety of areas of modern life.

While we owe respect and respect to the earliest techniques of breathing, which are still relevant modern approaches provide an exciting, new perspective. Modern methods are based on the earlier methods and have developed new techniques that have created entirely new concepts of breathwork and health.

In the final section, we will to learn about two of the most modern holistic breathwork techniques that are known by the names of SOMA Breath and the Wim Hof Method. They provide a comprehensive review of breathwork and provide an integrated view of breathwork that addresses the mental and physical wellbeing of both.

Alongside describing the fundamental features of these innovative methods, we'll also explore the ways in which they have built on tradition-based knowledge and will draw attention to the various contributions they have made to the field of mindful breathing.

SOMA Breath: A Energized Meditation

Traditional Pranayama practice is a way to identify a variety of goals to master the breath. These include clarity, clarity, and spiritual advancement. The SOMA Breath technique is much more simple in its primary goal to help you achieve real happiness.

The SOMA Breath was founded with Niraj Naik, the SOMA Breath community was founded by Niraj Naik, and a method for holistic breathing. The SOMA Breath method incorporates elements of yoga, Pranayama, holistic health mindfulness eating, and most importantly music. In contrast to traditional breathing practices that tries to block out the noise around us music is an essential component of this SOMA method. It was specifically designed for this purpose that it serves, it is SOMA Breath music helps to improve concentration and helps to create greater connection to the consciousness.

Instead of solely looking at the breathing process it is a more holistic approach. SOMA Breath is based on an approach that is community-based and develops specific plans for each person. There are many benefits associated with this breath, for example, decreasing stress levels, increasing physical and mental endurance and reducing the rate of breathing and reducing inflammation in addition to many others. (About SOMA Breath and Niraj Naik, n.d.).

The focus is on holistic multidisciplinary healing that is scientifically based and that blends the best lessons from various fields of mindfulness to achieve the highest outcomes. According to the site, "SOMA Breath, considered as a whole, and with its variety of uses and applications, provides an instrument for life-long change" (About SOMA Breath & Niraj Naik, n.d.).

Contrary to the particular techniques we've previously discussed as a way to incorporate within a busy routine without requiring a major life-style change, this approach is geared towards different aspects of life and the various levels of consciousness. It seeks to bring mindfulness and clarity to all aspects of existence, from practical considerations, like the best food choices is best to feed our bodies as well as more profound questions, such as how to manage our insanity. The main strength of SOMA is in the holistic re-examination of health The SOMA approach can, in turn be viewed as a form of lifestyle that demands a more profound commitment.

Many practitioners have been awed by Naik's techniques, and have confirmed the transformative impact that it has had on their lives. From dealing with difficult situations, to strengthening an existing meditation practice, and even achieving higher levels of awareness and awakening, SOMA Breath seems to deliver the promises it makes.

Wim Hof Breathing Method

Wim Hof Method Wim Hof Method is another contemporary approach to breathing which, like SOMA Breath, SOMA Breath, aims to find ways to integrate breathwork into an holistic approach to health. It is a holistic approach to wellness. Wim Hof Method offers a distinct approach to holistic wellness and is focused on regaining control of the physical mechanisms of our body , and tap into our inner potential.

Perhaps you've been aware about Wim Hof often referred to by the name "The Iceman." Hof has broken numerous records by enduring extreme cold and exercising vigorously under extreme conditions. According Hof, according to Hof the key to his incredible endurance is the practice of what he calls the Wim Hof Method (WHM) A series of breathing exercises and exposure that are designed to help us reconnect with nature and to unlock our potential.

According to self-reported accounts, this method is associated with improved levels of energy, decreased depression and anxiety symptoms, greater focus and a greater feeling of self-relation (Allen 2018,). In this article we will go over the fundamental principles of this method , and we will also explore the breathing technique that is associated with it.

According to the WHM website the three elements for this practice including the use of breathing, cold therapy and the commitment to a regular routine (Hof, n.d.). The exposure to cold temperatures offers certain benefits, including decreasing inflammation and the tension in muscles and pain, especially for athletes with high intensity. There are, however, some health risks that come with it so it's best to take it slow and seek approval from a medical professional prior to engaging in this activity.

Commitment The third principle of the WHM, is the concept that guides this technique. The increase in willpower is the primary benefit that is promised by practicing Wim Hof. This is achieved through regular meditation and reconnecting with the primal nature and staying consistent in the routine.

Breathwork practice is also a key component to this technique. The breathing technique devised by Wim Hof utilizes the combination of hyperventilation and anapnea and breathing in a controlled manner (Hof 2014).

Before learning the basic principles of breathing techniques Wim Hof invented, be sure that it's suitable for you to practice breathing exercises that involve hyperventilation or apnea. Similar to Kapalbhati and Kapalbhati, if you have

Diabetes, high blood pressure or heart issues, or are expecting, you might consider sitting this one out. Be aware of the signals your body may be sending you, and look out for signs of dizziness , or fatigue.

For the first time start by finding a sitting or lying position where you can be relaxed. Inhale deeply and exhale using your mouth. We want an increase in speed than normal breathing but not as quick or forceful as when you breathe of fire. Make sure you're fully breathing in through the chest and stomach and exhaling completely through your mouth. It is recommended to be taking between 30 to 40 long, powerful, energizing breaths each session.

Following this initial round in deep oxygenation we're going to keep the breath the length of time that is comfortable. Begin with a brief period and then increase the duration as you get more comfortable with. The hold can be interrupted for a breath deep and then hold the breath in for a further 15 seconds or for as long as is to be comfortable. The oxygenation that you received from the previous exercise will help you hold your breath a bit easier. Then exhale completely.

The exercise set is one exercise. Hof suggests repeating the exercise at least three times with no interruption prior to completing the workout (Hof 2014). The practice will make you feel more energetic and more focused. it will help you achieve the ideal mental state to meditate.

People who practice the WHM have seen life-changing changes within a couple of sessions, such as conquering deep-seated fears, improving self-esteem, and alleviating chronic back problems. Similar to the SOMA method, this approach is a commitment to a adjustments to lifestyles, and therefore isn't the most lasting introduction to breathing for someone who is new to. However, we can implement some of its concepts to our everyday lives, and use the breathing method to achieve an energy boost.

Chapter 9: Breath Work To Treat Anxiety

"Anxiety will not completely fill tomorrow with its sadness, but it only empty today of its power." -- Charles Spurgeon

Feeling anxious thoughts and fears is an everyday aspect of life. The prospect of a job interview and an unpaid bill an appointment with a new person or a project that has failed or health concerns are just a few aspects of everyday life that could trigger anxiety. They can manifest physically, like sweaty palms or anxiety and tension in the muscles. With all the negative consequences of worrying on our body as well as the mind and heart, it's easy to suggest, "just stop worrying," but it's not always easy.

What is anxiety?

The sweaty palms and muscles, tension and feelings of anxiety are all indications the body may be in tension and that the stress hormone is activated. The anxiety you cannot manage to eliminate is known as anxiety. Anxiety is your body's normal response to stress. it can make people feel anxious or fearful. Stress and anxiety are a part of daily life. But, when the signs of anxiety get severe, it should be considered a reason to be concerned. If you notice that these symptoms are hindering normal mental, physical and emotional functions, or last for more than six month, it is possible that the person experiencing the problem is suffering from an anxiety disorder.

Anxiety Disorders

Anxiety-related symptoms are normal and can be temporary, but don't hinder your from taking part in your daily life. Anxiety disorders, on contrary, are characterized by intense emotions and painful. These emotions prevent you from doing what you enjoy and from going to the places you'd like to visit. The anxiety can be so intense that it stops the person suffering from leaving their home or even crossing the street because of fear.

Here's a list common anxiety disorders and how they manifest.

* Agoraphobia. The anxiety condition is defined by an extreme avoidance of certain places or situations that can make sufferers feel scared or helpless. or even embarrassed.

111

* Body-focused repetitive behavior. They are a set of routine behaviors that sufferers engage in to combat constant anxiety. These can include lips biting, hair pulling and picking at the skin.

A general anxiety disorder. It is characterized by persistent and frequent anxiety about events or activities which are insignificant to the event or activity. It could also be the case in the context of everyday problems. This kind of anxiety disorder typically is seen together with other anxiety disorders or mental disorders like depression.

"Health Anxiety. This is a class of disorders that are defined by the patient experiencing one or more of the somatic signs of a pre-existing or developing illness or.

• Panic disorders. It is characterized by repeated bouts of panic and anxiety that are unexpected attacks that are result of intense anxiety. The panic attacks and feelings anxiety are often followed by a worry that they'll happen again, and the patient develops a pattern of trying to avoid the event or undertaking.

"Post-traumatic Stress Disorder. This anxiety disorder is an outcome of experiencing or witnessing an extreme trauma.

"Separation anxiety. This is a condition of anxiety that causes a person to experience an excessive fear of being separated from a particular individual, for example, a spouse or blood relation.

"Social anxiety" disorder. This is the condition which causes sufferers to feel extremely nervous when they are in social settings.

There are a lot of the many anxiety disorders that are present and require physician if symptoms continue to be present and make every day life difficult.

The causes of anxiety

The root of anxiety is not well recognized by the scientists. There are however common external factors that be a contributing factor to the development of anxiety. These comprise:

* Financial stress

• Side-effects of medications

* Stress that comes from emotional trauma such as the loss of a loved one or family member.

* Stress related to personal relationships, such as in the case of a romantic relationship.

• The usage of illegal substances like cocaine or heroin and withdrawal from these substances.

* Being a sign of a medical condition such as a heart attack.

It has been demonstrated that people who are susceptible to developing anxiety may be driven to develop anxiety disorders due to traumatic life events such as abuse or the loss of loved family members. There are other risk factors like genetics, alcohol and drug abuse as well as personality and trauma in childhood that make it more likely to develop chronic anxiety.

Signs of anxiety

Common signs of anxiety include:

* An increase in heart rate

* Breathing rapid (hyperventilation)

* Struggling to concentrate upon anything else than the actual tension

Feelings of fatigue or weakness

* Sweating

* Tense

* Headaches

* Irritability

Feelings of imminent disaster, panic, or fear

* Trouble falling asleep and being unable to fall asleep

* Suffering from gastrointestinal issues

Anxiety and. Stress

The two are frequently misunderstood because they share many of the similar symptoms. Some physical symptoms that they share are rapid blood pressure, muscular tension and headaches. Other symptoms might include fatigue, lack of concentration as well as sleeplessness, insomnia, and anxiety. With the many symptoms that they share it can be difficult to discern stress from anxiety however this section will help to eliminate the confusion.

It is a brief feeling that arises when triggered by a situation like an interview or nearly being struck by a car. It is often due to an external cause and is therefore treatable by eliminating these triggers from the environment in which the sufferer is. Stress doesn't need to be negative. It could be the motivation one needs to perform better in a particular situation. Stress is a source of negativity that causes issues such as sleeplessness and a diminished capability to accomplish the things that you do.

Anxiety On the other hand it is a condition that occurs suddenly that is caused by stress. Contrary to stress, which disappears out when the cause of stress is removed and anxiety may persist after. It can cause impairment in social, occupational and everyday functioning. The root in anxiety can be internal which makes it harder to deal with. Since the issue is internalized, it's often difficult to determine the root cause, which is a further aspect to the difficulty of receiving the proper treatment.

How to release anxiety through Breathing

As previously mentioned stress, and consequently anxiety-induced chest breathing which triggers the release cortisol, which triggers the body into fight-or-flight mode. This causes a disruption in the balance of oxygen entering the body, and carbon dioxide that leaves the body. This imbalance causes increasing frequency of anxiety and panic attacks. If you are able to bring your breathing in check and restoring the equilibrium, you can in reducing stress and anxiety. Here are some breathing techniques that you can use to fight anxiety.

Breathing via the Diaphragm

Be aware that breathing through the diaphragm helps balance the intake of oxygen and carbon dioxide elimination and also helps keep your mind at ease. In order to ensure you are breathing the diaphragm, not your chest, make sure that you're sitting or lying in a comfortable posture with your neck, shoulders as well as your head in a comfortable posture. Be sure the knees of your feet are bent. Then, put a hand beneath your ribs and place the other on your chest. Inhale with your nose and exhale through your pursed lips. Make sure that your belly moves greater than the chest when you breathe in and exhale. This can be done for up to 10 minutes, approximately three times per day.

Breaths with Focused Breaths

A slow, deep breathing pattern that is steady and focused helps to reduce anxiety. Begin by sitting down on a couch or lying in a neutral, secure setting. Breathe normally in and out and then observe how your body feels while you breathe. This lets you discover the areas of tension within your body.

Then, exhale deeply and slowly breathe through your nose. Be sure to expand your belly over your chest while you inhale. Inhale slowly, and sigh as you like. The tension will be released. you feel. Keep doing this for as long as you like and be aware of the rising and falling of your stomach. While inhaling, think the sensation of being swept away by waves of tranquility. Think that all negative thoughts or energies you carry in your body are being cleansed every moment you exhale. Be sure not to be distracted by this process to maximize the effect.

The Exhale that is Lengthened

Deep breaths during anxiety attacks could make the attack since inhales are connected to the sympathetic nerve system, which regulates the fight-or-flight response. However exhaling triggers the parasympathetic nervous system. which aids in relaxing the body. Inhaling fast and often can result in hyperventilation particularly in a stressful situation. Thus, conscious lengthening of your breath can help to reduce anxiety and ease your mind.

To do this, push the air out of your lungs in counts of six while inhaling for counts of four. This makes your exhale slightly longer than your inhales. Do this for 2 to 5 minutes while seated or lying in a comfortable position in a neutral, calm environment.

Lion's Breath

This breathing exercise expands on the one outlined above by promoting exhaling forcefully. The practice gets its name from the fierce lion-like expression on the practitioner's face during exhales. The pose used and the rhythm of breathing are well-known in the yogi community to reduce anger, stress and anxiety.

To practice the lion's breath, get into a kneeling position in a safe, calm environment. Ensure that your ankles are crossed and that your behind is resting on your feet. If the kneeling position is uncomfortable for you, sit cross-legged.

As you bring your hands to your knees and stretch out your arms and fingers, breathe in through your nose then out through your mouth as you vocalize a short sound. While you exhale, open your mouth as wide as you can and stick your tongue out as far down as it can go. Focus on the end of your nose or the middle of your forehead as you exhale.

Relax your face when you inhale. Repeat the entire process six times. Change the cross of your ankles halfway through the process.

Equal Breathing

This breathing technique stems from the ancient practice of pranayama yoga, and it involves inhaling for the same amount of time that you exhale. This balance helps to reduce anxiety. Begin the breathing exercise by ensuring that you are lying or sitting down in a position that you are comfortable. Do this in a safe and calm environment. Close your eyes and breathe normally. Pay attention to what is going on in your body and locate the tension. Inhale through your nose and slowly count to four. Next, exhale and do the same slow count to four. As you continue to repeat this inhale and exhale process, be mindful of the feelings in your body and the sense of fullness and emptiness in your lungs as you breathe.

Resonate Breathing

This breathing technique is also called coherent breathing. It helps induce a relaxed state and calms anxiety. To begin, lie down and close your eyes in a neutral, safe environment. With your mouth closed, breathe in gently through your nose for a count of six. Do not overfill your lungs with air. Next, exhale for six seconds. Gently allow the air to leave your body. Continue this process for up to 10 minutes. In this time, you should notice that your heart rate mimics the calm rhythm of your breathing. This breathing technique is so effective at reducing anxiety because it helps synchronize breath with heart rate, which aids in the balance of oxygen coming into the body and carbon dioxide leaving.

Alternate Nostril Breathing

This breathing technique is a great one for improving mental focus and concentration as well as reducing anxiety as it facilitates the provision of equal amounts of oxygen to the brain while expelling carbon dioxide in the same quantity.

Meditation to Reduce Anxiety

In addition to employing the breathing techniques outlined above to fight anxiety, you can make use of meditation to help alleviate the symptoms.

What is Meditation?

There has been some confusion about what meditation is. Before I explain what it is, let's take a moment to discuss what it is not.

Meditation is not about making yourself evolve into a new, different, or even better person. While you practice meditation, the purpose is not to turn off your feelings or thoughts. Meditation is not a religion.

Instead, meditation is a technique that allows the mind to become inwardly focused, clear, and relaxed so that it functions more efficiently. Meditation is a continual process that helps retrain your brain to process thoughts and feelings in new ways. Meditation relies on principles and science that allow the practitioner to gain a new awareness of themselves as well as a sense of perspective. All of this is aimed at enabling them to understand himself or herself better.

This newfound awareness leads to being more mindful. Mindfulness is the ability that a person develops so that they can be present in each moment and fully engaged in whatever activity they are doing. Mindfulness teaches you to recognize harmful and self-defeating thought patterns and behaviors so that you can steer yourself onto a more constructive course.

To manage and reduce anxiety, the first thing that is needed is an understanding of what is triggering it and how it operates.

Meditation allows for inward reflection and understanding. Anxiety comes from the inability to regulate your emotions internally, and meditation helps reprogram the pathways in the brain that help this regulation hence improving one's personal ability to control their emotions so an anxiety attack can be prevented. Meditation allows you to familiarize yourself with the thoughts and feelings that induce anxiety within you. By becoming familiar with these triggers, you can release yourself from their grip because you will realize that these thoughts and feelings do not define you or your reactions to them.

With the self-awareness that comes with meditation, you will also become conscious of what your body is feeling in each moment including during an anxiety attack. This allows you to become more prepared and even better able to stop anxiety before it even starts.

Benefits of Meditation

The benefits of meditation extended far and wide and supported by science. While of course, you can use meditation to help relieve stress, reduce anxiety and get peace of mind, there are many more physical, emotional and mental benefits that should encourage you to continue practicing meditation. These benefits include:

• Reduced risk of developing cardiovascular diseases. Since there is a reduction in stress levels when you practice meditation, stress hormones are not released into the bloodstream, so heart rate and blood pressure remain balanced. This balance keeps your heart healthy and in good working order which lowers the risk of developing cardiovascular diseases such as heart attack and stroke.

• Increased energy levels. A significant part of proper meditation is controlling your breath. This ensures that oxygen and carbon dioxide levels remain balanced in the body, which allows it to stay calm and relaxed. With a proper balance of oxygen and carbon dioxide in the body, red blood cells remain properly oxygenated, leading to higher levels of energy.

● Better immunity. Decreased levels of stress and anxiety mean that the body is better able to fight off diseases. The body often inadvertently attacks itself under stressful and anxious conditions. With lowered stress and anxiety levels, the body can better regulate its immune responses.

● Better sleep. Reduced stress and anxiety levels allow the body to fall into a restful state easier, resulting in better quality and adequate quantity of sleep.

● Better emotional health. A side effect of stress and anxiety is decreased self-image and a negative outlook on life, which can lead to depression. The hormones that are released during stress and anxiety can also negatively affect the sufferer's mood. Meditation allows the practitioner to become aware of these emotions and therefore, to better control them so that they can gain a more positive and happier outlook on life.

More benefits of meditation include lengthened attention span, increased memory, concentration, focus, increased self-compassion and kindness toward others, aiding in fighting addictions as well as pain relief.

A Simple Mindful Meditation Exercise

While a meditation exercise can go on for hours, all that is needed, especially for a beginner, is a commitment of 5 to 30 minutes each day. Most people find that just 15 minutes every day is ideal. Try to do this at the same time in the same location every day so that you build a habit. Eventually, you will not have to think about doing it. Your body will go through the motions automatically.

There are several types of meditation. They include:

- Mindful meditation
- Moving meditation

- Mantra meditation

- Body scanning meditation

- Visualization meditation

- Gazing meditation

There are other types as well. Each type of meditation has its benefits, but we will focus on mindful meditation in this section. Mindful meditation involves using the breath to focus the attention of the meditation practitioner. This type of meditation relies on keeping your mind focused on the present. Your mind should not wander to the past or what you have going on in the next few minutes. You need to be still, relaxed and allow your brain and heart to heal internally. This means that you need to keep your mind from wandering or being distracted. You can keep your eyes closed to help with this, but it is not necessary if you are more comfortable with them open. If you would prefer to close your eyes but find it hard to do, try an eye mask.

If you are a newbie, staying focused will be hard to accomplish. Do not fret! When you notice your mind is starting to wander, simply refocus on your breath and bring yourself back to the present moment.

For mindful meditation to be most effective, do it in a distraction-free zone with ample time. This will let you concentrate on clearing your mind and following the rhythm of your breath. This can be anytime that is convenient for you. That may be early in the more, late at night or even on your lunch hour.

Before you start, get comfortable. Put on loose, soft clothing and unwind in your favorite way. Doing a few light stretches while listening to tranquil, soothing music can help you achieve this relaxed mindset.

Try this simple mindful meditation you can do in the comfort of your own home at any time.

1.   Sit or lie down in a comfortable position. There is no set rule about what position you should take, only that you can

stay in that position for some time and remain comfortable. If you choose to sit, ensure that you are not slouching and your spine is straight. Remain relaxed and put your hands on your lap. If you sit on the floor, the recommended position is cross-legged. If you sit in a chair, ensure that your feet are resting on the floor.

2.   Breathe in and out slowly. Start by taking a few slow and deep breaths while you inhale through your nose and exhale through your mouth. The first few breaths are likely to be shallow but as you continue, ensure that you fill your lungs each time so that your breaths become deeper. This will make you feel calmer and more relaxed. Do not force the breathing process because this will make you tense up and defy the purpose of this practice. As you breathe, pay attention to the movement of your body such as how your belly moves, how your shoulders move up and down, how the air feels passing through your nose, etc. Pay attention to how you feel and the musings of your mind. Keep present in the moment and if

your mind wanders, bring it back to the breath.

3.   Open your eyes after 15 minutes have passed and move from your position.

That is it! This simple, 3-step procedure can help you reduce anxiety and many other benefits.

Guided meditation is also effective at reducing anxiety because it interrupts the pattern of thinking that facilitates stress and therefore, anxiety. Guided meditation is led by a third party which can be a yoga instructor, an audio recording or even yourself giving instructions. The third-party leads you with instructions on how to relax specific muscles in your body and with visualizations so that you get the most benefit from the meditation exercise. The added benefit of guided meditation is that someone else is there to keep you focused so that your mind does not wander. Guided meditation also offers direction and gives you a voice you can focus on during the exercise.

Chapter 10: Breath Work For Anger

Management

"Every day we have plenty of opportunities to get angry, stressed or offended. But what you're doing when you indulge these negative emotions is giving something outside yourself power over your happiness. You can choose to not let little things upset you." – Joel Osteen

What is Anger?

Everyone feels anger but how we deal with it is what defines us.

Anger is a powerful emotion that results from feeling hurt, frustrated, disappointed, or annoyed. Anger can vary in intensity from mild irritation to intense rage and fury. Both internal and external triggers can cause irritation. External triggers can be someone cutting you off in traffic or your boss, giving you another task at the end of an already long workday. Internal triggers might be memories of traumatic or enraging events.

Signs of anger can include:

- Grinding the teeth or clenching the jaw
- Sweating
- Trembling or shaking
- Increased and rapid heart rate
- Rapid, shallow breathing
- Increased blood pressure
- Muscle tension
- Stomach ache
- Headache
- Dizziness
- Feeling warm around the face and neck
- Feeling emotions such as sadness, guilt, resentment, and irritation
- Feeling overwhelmed
- Feeling anxious

133

- Feeling the need to strike out in a physical or verbal way

- Feeling like you need to get away from the situation

In extreme cases, signs of anger may include acting in an abrasive or abusive manner, yelling, screaming, crying or craving a substance to help relax.

Myths about Anger

Anger itself is not a bad thing. It is an entirely reasonable human emotion. That might surprise you to read, but there are many other misconceptions about anger circulating out there, including this one. Let's take a moment to help clear up the confusion by looking at these myths about anger.

Myth #1 - Anger is a negative emotion.

Anger is not a negative emotion, and it is very healthy that you feel it now and then. Feelings of anger can lead to positive change because it is only through feeling anger that we get up and do something. Was an injustice done to someone in your community, and you felt the need to do something about it? If your answer is yes, then a positive outcome can stem from your anger. Many laws have been passed because a large enough group felt angry about an injustice and did something about it.

Myth #2 - Anger is all in your head.

That is incorrect because you feel anger physically, emotionally, and mentally. Your face gets flushed, your body shakes, your heart rate picks up, you feel the urge to hit something, you feel betrayed. These are signs that have to do with more than just your mental process, and are all the result of anger.

Myth #3 - Anger and aggression are the same things.

They certainly are not. While anger can lead to positive change, merely reacting does not bode well for anyone. Aggressive behavior is unhealthy and can damage others, including the person who is angry in physical, emotional, and mental ways.

While anger can be felt involuntarily, acting out is a choice.

Myth #4 - Ignoring anger makes it go away.

Smiling to cover up your anger or denying your feelings is called suppression and suppression of anger is unhealthy as it disturbs your peace of mind and can make you direct that anger inward. Suppressed anger has been linked to several physical and mental health problems, such as depression and hypertension. Also, suppressed anger can erupt and manifest as aggressive and abusive behavior. Finding a healthy outlet and calmly expressing your anger works a lot better.

Myth #5 - Men get angrier than women.

This is false. Men and women have the same propensity to feel anger. The difference lies in that men are more likely to show aggressive and compulsive expressions to the anger compared to women.

Myth #6 - Anger management classes and therapy do not work.

This is false. Most of the time, there are negative consequences in response to anger; it is because people do not know how to handle their emotions well. Anger management classes and therapy offer persons with anger issues, especially those who have aggressive outbursts, tools, and techniques that can help them better manage their emotions and thus, their response to anger.

Anger can be a force for positive change, or it can have a negative outcome. It all depends on how the person chooses to handle it and react to it.

Anger Disorders

Anger disorders are a pattern of behavior that includes pathological aggression and violent behaviors that are a symptom of and driven by an underlying and chronically repressed anger or rage. Most people who exhibit signs of an anger disorder have a history of mismanagement of anger, including anger suppression. This mismanagement often leads to resentment, bitterness, hatred, and rage. Anger disorders are often a symptom of other disorders like OCD and ADHD, both of which will be discussed in the next section. Substance abuse can also lead to anger disorders.

The most commonly known anger disorder is called Intermittent Explosive Disorder (IED). Sudden episodes of unwarranted anger characterize this disorder. People who suffer from this disorder describe it as losing control of their emotions and being overcome by anger. This loss of control impairs their judgment, and they may threaten or attack people, animals and objects. This disorder is normally diagnosed after a person has displayed at least three episodes of aggressive outbursts that show a lack of apparent provocation or reason.

There are a variety of factors that may lead to IED. They include genetics. While no specific gene has been located to be associated with the disorder, there has been a trend shown in families. There has also been research that indicates abnormalities in areas of the brain regulate inhibition. This abnormality can lead to impulsive violent behavior.

Environment also plays in the development of this anger disorder. Children who grow up exposed to a person with IED or who have been subjected to harsh treatment at the hands of someone in authority are likely to develop IED at an early age.

Other factors that can lead to developing IED include:

- Experiencing emotional trauma
- Experiencing physical trauma
- Some medical conditions
- A history of substance abuse
- Being male

In addition to the normal signs of anger, a person with IED can also exhibit these other symptoms:

- Physical and verbal aggression

- Damaging property

- Road rage

- Angry outbursts

- Physically attacking people, animals, and objects

- Low frustration tolerance

- Brief periods of emotional detachment

The effects of IED are far-reaching and do not only affect the sufferer. The effects that IED can have include:

- Legal issues

- Imprisonment

- Drug and alcohol abuse and addiction

- Impaired interpersonal relationships

- Trouble concentrating and focusing at home, work and school

- Low self-esteem and self-confidence

- Domestic and child abuse

- Self-harm

- Suicidal thoughts and behaviors

If you or someone you know suffers from an anger disorder, I urge you to seek help from a medical practitioner such as a therapist so that you can get the assistance you need before you do irreversible damage to yourself or others.

Causes of Anger Disorders

Anger can have several causes. These include:

- Depression. Along with the other symptoms that occur over an extended period of at least two weeks, sadness and loss of interest are often felt along with anger in this condition. This anger may be outwardly expressed and visible to others, but other times it is suppressed.

- Grief. Grief is defined as deep sorrow. There are several stages to the process of grief which can come as a result of a breakup, losing a job, the death of a loved one and more. Including anger, there are five stages of grief. The other four stages are denial, bargaining, depression, and acceptance. The anger that the grieving person will feel may be directed inward or outward.

• Alcohol abuse. Alcohol abuse, also known as alcoholism, refers to the consumption of too much alcohol at one time as well as regular use. It impairs the drinker's ability to think coherently and to make rational decisions. It has also been shown that drinking alcohol increases instances of aggression, which is a symptom of anger.

• Drug abuse. Just as with alcohol abuse, one of the consequences of drug abuse, such as heroin and cocaine abuse, is aggressive behavior which is a sign of anger.

• Traumatic experiences. Traumatic experiences, such as abuse and childhood trauma, often trigger anger and violent outbursts due to uncontrollable emotions. Anger is a coping mechanism to help this person deal with the negativity they experienced, but this anger is self-destructive. People who get angry for this reason often need the assistance of a medical practitioner such as a therapist to work through this.

• Obsessive-Compulsive Disorder. Also referred to as OCD, Obsessive-Compulsive Disorder is an anxiety disorder that is characterized by compulsive behavior and obsessive thoughts. OCD is characterized by disturbing thoughts, urges, and images that make a person do something repetitively. Anger is often a symptom of OCD because the person becomes frustrated with the inability to prevent the obsessive thoughts and behaviors.

• Attention Deficit Hyperactivity Disorder. Also known as ADHD, this is a neurodevelopmental disorder that includes symptoms such as impulsivity, hyperactivity, and inattention. These symptoms are often exhibited in early childhood and continue throughout a person's life. Anger is a symptom of ADHD.

• Bipolar disorder. This is a disorder that causes dramatic and intense shifts in mood. Anger is one of the intense emotions that a person who has bipolar disorder will feel.

● Oppositional Defiant Disorder. Sometimes referred to as ODD, this is a disorder that results in defiant and angry behavior toward authority. While this disorder is most common in children, it is also seen in adults.

What is Anger Management?

The natural way to express anger, which was passed down from early caveman, is with aggression. Anger is an adaptive response that helps human beings eliminate threats to themselves. It invokes feelings of power as well, which is why it can become addictive. In essence, anger was necessary for survival.

However, we have come a long way from our ancestors and do not need to lash out aggressively to assert dominance or state our position in a situation. We evolved and learned to express our feelings calmly throughout the history of civilization.

It can still be difficult to suppress our instincts. As seen from the number of disorders that exhibit anger as a symptom, anger is not something that a person can always control or avoid. You can, however, learn to control your reaction. The first step in effectively managing your anger is learning to recognize the signs when you are angry. These have been listed above. You should familiarize yourself with them so that you know what to look out for. Next, you can employ strategies to manage your anger in a safe, effective way

Anger management is the process of learning to recognize that you are angry then taking proactive measures to calm down and deal with the situation that is productively angering you. There are classes and therapy available if you need help to diffuse anger. If you suffer from issues like ADHD and depression, there are also medications that your medical practitioner can prescribe to help you if needed. However, there are simple strategies that you can employ alone or in addition to the advice you receive from your doctor, in class or therapy and the effects of any medication.

You can find some of these strategies to help defuse your anger below.

Visualize yourself being calm

Calming your anger starts in your mind. Manifest a calmer, more relaxed state by imagining that you are in that state. It helps to remove yourself temporarily from the situation that is making you angry. Find a quiet place to sit, close your eyes and let your imagination show you a calm and happy version of yourself. Include the small details in your mental imagery such as what it feels like, what your facial expressions look like and even what you smell in that moment.

Remove yourself from the situation

Take a timeout. If a situation is increasing your anger level, remove yourself from it so that you can calm down and think clearly. Then, you can figure out how to handle the situation in a more productive way.

Count to 10

If you cannot remove yourself from the angering situation, you can still calm yourself down. Close your eyes if you must and slowly count to 10. As you could imagine a wave of calm washing over you. This will afford you at least 10 seconds to control your emotions and therefore, your behavior.

Think before you speak

We are often tempted to lash out when we are angry. This includes verbally. In this time, we tend to say things we do not mean or did not mean to say at that time. To avoid this verbal vomit, take a few moments to detach yourself from the situation and hold your tongue until you have calmed down.

Progressive muscle relaxation

Muscle tension is a sign of anger. By encouraging your muscles to relax, you can diffuse your anger. One method of encouraging muscle relaxation is called progressive muscle relaxation. This is often applied to different parts of the body one area at a time. For example, a relaxation technique you can apply to your abdomen is gently tightening the muscles of your stomach as you inhale. Keep from straining your muscles. As you do this, you will notice the tension. Release the tense as you exhale and pay attention to the way your muscles relax in response. Repeat this for 2 minutes. As you pay attention to the tensed and relaxed states of your muscles, you can work to bring them to a permanently relaxed state. You can then move onto another body area such as the chest and shoulders and repeat the same technique.

Exercise

Exercise and physical activities like dancing, help reduce stress, tension, and anxiety by activating the release of feel-good hormones and promoting deep breathing. This helps maintain the oxygen intake, carbon dioxide release balance. These conditions also help reduce anger as well as help you improve your mood. It is great to make this a habit but developing a schedule such as working out three mornings a week. When an action becomes a habit, it will not feel like such a chore to do. Developing a habit for exercise and physical activity is especially important if you are a person who does not like to do.

Get a support system

Try to maintain relationships with people that you can have meaningful conversations with. In that way, you can talk about your feelings and these people will help you see things from a different point of view. Understanding from another point of view can help reduce your anger. This also helps keep you from feeling isolated. Having a support system lightens the emotional load, which makes it more bearable and therefore, easier to control.

Keep a journal

In addition to talking out your feelings so that you can gain a different point of view and find closure to help reduce your anger, you can write them down. You can keep a journal, which can be a simple notebook. By writing your thoughts and feelings down, you can examine them closer and revisit them when you are more level headed so that you can better understand what triggers your anger. This might be the turning point that allows you better control over your emotions.

Try to find humor in the situation

Laughter usually makes things better, and that list includes anger. Try to find something to laugh about in the heat of the moment. Laughter and smiling (even forced laughter and fake smiles) release more of those feel-good hormones, which elevates the mood and reduces anger.

Practice listening

Anger often arises because of miscommunication between people. Communication is the process of one party, sending a message to be interpreted by another party. Communication is only effective if the latter party receives and understands the message as it was intended. Active listening is part of proper communication. Improving your listening skills can help you communicate better. You may find that you are no longer so easy to anger because of this.

Control the way you breath

One of the most effective natural methods of controlling anger is by learning to breathe your way through it. This is explained more in-depth below.

How to Cope With Anger through Breathing

As you might have noted, one of the symptoms of anger is rapid, shallow breathing. This forces you to breathe through your chest rather than your diaphragm. This has all the usually internal reactions such as an imbalance of oxygen intake and carbon dioxide release and the release of stress hormones. One of the ways to control your anger is by slowing and deepening your breath.

To ensure that whatever breathing exercise that you practice is effective, try to find a quiet, comfortable place. This can be in your bed, in your car or even while you sit on the toilet. The location does not matter. What matters is that you have a distraction-free neutral and comforting place to practice. You also need to ensure that you are relaxed and your muscles are at ease. Use the progressive muscle relaxation technique to release any tenseness. Pay attention to your facial features as well, and notice the way they react when you inhale and exhale.

While you can, of course, try breathing exercises in the heat of the moment to calm your anger and feelings of rage, you can also practice breathing for anger daily so you become more mindful and self-aware. This allows you to control yourself better when you are angry rather than having to deal with the fallout of a negative reaction.

Some of the breathing techniques that we have already discussed in previous chapters also help with reducing anger. They include:

- Lion's breath

- Focused breaths

- Breathing through the diaphragm

- 4-7-8 breathing technique

Also, here are a few more breathing techniques that can help you overcome the intensity of your anger. Some of these include yoga poses that are highly concentrated on breathwork.

Complete Breath

This breathing technique concentrates on imagery as it allows you to picture the negativity that builds as a result of anger leaving your body with every exhale. To do it, sit cross-legged with your spine straight. Inhaling deeply and slowly, bringing your breath into your diaphragm. Place your hand over your chest and allow your ribcage to rise with this inhale. Hold this pose for three counts then exhale completely and imagine that your negative thoughts and emotions leave your body with the air. Repeat until you feel purged those negative thoughts and emotions.

Breathing for Relaxation

As the title suggests, this breathing technique is used for getting into a state of relaxation. It can also be used to blow away anger, stress, and anxiety. For relaxation, lie on your back in a comfortable position and allow your body to drain of all tension. Place your right hand on your chest and your left hand over your abdomen. Breathe deeply and let your natural rhythm take over. Your inhales and exhales should equate to the same amount of time. As you inhale and exhale, allow only your left-hand rise and fall. Your right hand should remain motionless.

Corpse Pose

This yoga pose is great for calming the body and mind as well as allowing the practitioner to focus on the natural rhythmic state of them breathing, which aids in relaxation. To do this pose, lie on your back with your arms relaxed at your sides. Your palms should be facing up. Allow your feet to fall open comfortably. Breathe in and out through your nose and allow the air to pass through your diaphragm. Let the natural rhythm of your breathing take over and concentrate on the sound of air entering and leaving your body until you feel completely relaxed. Do not allow your mind to wander, and if it does bring it back to the present moment and re-concentrate on the sound of your breathing.

Child's Pose

This yoga pose is said to be wonderful for strengthening the connection between the mind and body and for keeping you in touch with how you feel. This is great for allowing you to handle your anger in a productive and come manner. To get into this pose, kneel on all fours on a comfortable mat. Bring your arms around to the sides of your body as you push back and allow your head to rest on the floor. Reach your arms out in front of you to extend your shoulders for an extended child's pose.

Other Forms of Meditation for Anger

Consistently and repeatedly practicing meditation allows the practitioner to better control and cope with their negative emotions such as anger. This management and control allow them to react to the anger in a way that they wish rather than just going with the ebb and flow of the emotion. By practicing meditation, you learn to respond to anger rather than react to it. There is a science to how this works, and here it is. Meditation encourages the practitioner to enter a mindful and self-aware state. This instantly calms the person and lowers their stress levels. This has the effect of lowering the production of cortisol. This magnifies the calm of the mind and increases focus and clarity. When your mind is calm, you are less likely to become angry. In this way, you learn to make rational decisions even in situations that would have otherwise angered you and triggered you to react without thought.

Meditation is a practice that relies on breathing techniques, and as such, it allows sufficient oxygen to enter the blood and travel to the brain for optimal performance. Meditation also promotes elevated moods, which increases the production of feel-good hormones in the body. When you feel happy, you are less likely to become angry.

Meditation also allows you to rewire the way that you think and behave during certain situations, even in times of anger. We all develop habits in response to certain situations and emotions, including anger. Some of these habits in response to anger may be lashing out verbally. Meditation allows you to think more clearly and to effectively let go of these bad habits so that you do not act out in an undesirable manner. Since meditation will enable you to balance your emotions better and to think more rationally, you can review the situation that may have provoked your anger from a different perspective and see a way out of it that is easy for everyone involved. Meditation really can be a game-changer in allowing you to react to anger in a productive, safe, and friendly way.

Here is a simple, 20-minute meditation exercise you can practice daily to help you calm your emotions and your mind for better anger management.

1.   In a quiet comfortable room, sit in a cross-legged position.

2.   Gently rest your hands on your thighs with your palms up. Pull your shoulders back and pay attention to the sensations in your body.

3.   You have the choice of keeping your eyes open or closing them. If you choose to keep your eyes open, try not to become distracted during this 20-minute session.

4.   Focus inward on your navel. Begin to breathe slowly and deeply through your

diaphragm. Every time you inhale or exhale count from one to ten, then back down to one. Every time you inhale, hold on to the tension at that location at your navel. Every time that you exhale release that tension with your breath

5.   Repeat this five times.

6.   Now, it is time to visualize an incident that triggered your anger. Allow yourself to picture the details and acknowledge your anger by saying, "I am angry." Repeat the statement ten times. Vary the pitch of your voice every time that you say it, such as in a louder, softer, faster, and then slower tone.

7.   Allow yourself to check for any other emotions that you felt during the incident that angered you. Once you have identified the emotion, again say this out loud in varying pitches. For example, you may say, "I feel embarrassed."

8.   Concentrate on your breath once more and every time that you exhale, imagine that you exhale that negative

emotion. Resume counting from 1 to 10 and back down to one until the 20-minute period is over.

9.   Allow yourself to stay present and do not concentrate on any particular thought once you have settled the angering issue in your mind. If your thoughts start to interrupt your counting, refocus on your breath, and count again from one.

The exercise is as simple as that, but after those 20 minutes, you should feel a lot calmer and more relaxed, especially if you had experienced anger directly before this. The exercise allowed you to relive the moment but to then react calmly to it and to gain relaxation. This builds the muscle memory of how you should respond in the moment of anger.

Chapter 11: Breath Work For Trauma

"Even in times of trauma, we try to maintain a sense of normality until we no longer can. That, my friends, is called surviving. Not healing. We never become whole again ... we are survivors. If you are here today... you are a survivor. But those of us who have made it thru hell and are still standing? We bare a different name: warriors." — Lori Goodwin

What is PTSD?

PTSD stands for Post-Traumatic Stress Disorder. This is a psychiatric disorder that occurs in people who have witnessed or experienced a traumatic event such as violent personal assault, acts of war, combat or a natural disaster. PTSD went by other names in the past such as shell shock during World War I, and combat fatigue after World War II. As a result, it is commonly associated with soldiers or older persons who have been through war such as veterans. But the fact is that PTSD does not only affect people who have been through warlike situations.

Anyone who has been through a type of traumatic experience can suffer the same symptoms of post-traumatic stress disorder. This psychiatric disorder is characterized by disturbing and intense thoughts and feelings that are related to the traumatic experience even long after the traumatic event has ended. These people often relive the traumatic event or experience through nightmares and flashbacks that cause extreme negative emotions like sadness, anger, and fear. This can also put a hole in the person's self-esteem, self-confidence, and their perceived self-worth.

As a result of this extreme emotional effect, persons with PTSD are often estranged from other people or feel detached from society since they typically like to avoid people and situations that could remind them of the traumatic event. Even if the person was not directly involved in the event or situation, PTSD can make it very difficult to resume a normal life. Something as simple as an unexpected noise or an accidental touch can trigger a flashback and the unsettling consequences that come with it. The symptoms of PTSD can be debilitating and interfere with the day-to-day functioning of the person who suffers from it. Therefore, getting effective treatment for PTSD symptoms is vital to resume normal function.

Symptoms of PTSD

PTSD symptoms often start soon after the traumatic event, such as within one month, but it is not unheard of for them to appear even years after the event.

PTSD does not just take a mental and emotional toll on the person suffering. There are physical ramifications, as well.

The symptoms of PTSD are placed in these four categories:

Avoidance Symptoms

This is characterized by the person who suffers from PTSD avoiding situations, people, and places that might trigger bad memories of their traumatic experience. Part of this avoidant technique may involve not speaking or thinking about the event at all. While the PTSD suffer might try to find relief from the troubling thoughts, feelings, and memories with avoidance, this is of no help since it prevents that person from confronting the event and therefore, moving past it to living a healthier, happier life. No matter how much this person tries to avoid the traumatic experience or reminders of it, it eventual resurfaces in their behavior patterns, thoughts, dreams, and more.

Intrusive Thoughts

This includes involuntary and repeated memories, flashbacks and distressing dreams that are centered around a traumatic event. Flashbacks can be severe and so vivid that a person feels like they are reliving the traumatic event and seen it before their very eyes. For example, if a person with PTSD is an army veteran and has a flashback to a shootout during wartime, he or she might not see or hear the crowd anymore. Instead, this person may become immersed in the events unfolding in their mind and react to the past memory rather than what is actually going on. Nightmares can even make this person reenact the traumatic events with actions such as sleepwalking and screaming while in the throws of a dream. This can also cause physical symptoms such as sweating and increased and rapid heartbeat.

Cognitive Symptoms

These symptoms include negative thoughts directed inward and outward. They affect how the person thinks and feels. As a result, this person may take to bashing themselves and their character. The effects also include feeling hopeless about the future, having memory problems like not remembering specific parts of the traumatic event, feeling guilt or shame over the event. It can also illicit the person to feel detached from friends, family and local community, or have difficulty maintaining close relationships. The activities or hobbies they once enjoyed leave them feeling emotionally numb and they will also experience difficulty in staying positive. Due to a negative mental environment, the person with PTSD is likely to develop a mental disorder such as depression and persistent anxiety. This person is also likely to shut themselves away socially, which makes PTSD and these other disorders all the harder to treat.

Hyperarousal Symptoms

This involves a high level of reactivity from the person living with PTSD. This includes changes in the physical and emotional reactions this person has. The changes are usually a stark difference compared to their reactions before they suffered the traumatic incident. These changes may include always being on guard, feeling in danger, trouble concentrating, trouble sleeping, feeling overwhelming often, feeling degrees of shame and guilt over the incident, exhibiting aggressive behavior and angry outbursts, being easily startled or frightened and exhibiting self-destructive behaviors such as alcoholism and driving too fast. Younger children may also show symptoms such as re-enacting the traumatic event or aspects of the traumatic event while they play and having thoughts and dreams that may not include elements of the traumatic event.

The intensity and combination of symptoms vary from person to person, and even from time to time. Some people may only exhibit PTSD symptoms when they are stressed while other people may need a trigger like a loud noise or being touched without permission. The symptoms of PTSD can be very severe, indeed. If you have PTSD and you find that the symptoms are getting worse or you have self-harm or suicidal thoughts, please get help right away. You can reach out to a trusted friend or colleague, contact a spiritual leader in your community, make an appointment with your doctor, mental health practitioner, or call the suicide hotline in your country.

Types of PTSD

There are five main types of PTSD. They are:

Acute Stress Disorder

The characteristics of this type of PTSD include mental confusion, disassociation, severe insomnia, being unable to assume basic self-care daily, and panicked reactions. Treatment for this includes removal from the scene of trauma, brief supportive psychotherapy, immediate support, and if needed medication to deal with anxiety insomnia and grief. This type of PTSD typically starts to exhibit symptoms within one month of the traumatic incident. The sufferer must exhibit symptoms for a minimum of 3 days to be diagnosed. The sufferer often re-experiences the traumatic event and therefore, tries to avoid reminders of that incident such as conversations, thoughts, places, and activities as much as possible. This person typically has trouble sleeping, is irritable, and has an exaggerated response.

Normal Stress Response

This occurs when a healthy adult has been exposed to a singular traumatic event in adulthood that inspires intense bad memories, feelings of unreality, distressing emotions, numbness, and cutting themselves off from relationships. A normal stress response is actually a precursor to full-blown PTSD and is typically experienced after something like an injury, accident, illness, or abandonment has occurred. Abnormal amounts of stress and tension lead to a normal stress response. Recover from this usually occurs within a few weeks when counseling is sought out. This counseling usually begins with the sufferer describing the traumatic events and the emotions that are related to events. Recovery is possible with education on how they can cope with the symptoms of PTSD.

Uncomplicated PTSD

Uncomplicated PTSD is a result of a person experiencing a singular major traumatic event rather than a series of traumatic events. This fact makes it easier to treat. This type of PTSD is characterized by persistent re-experiencing of the traumatic event, emotional numbness, symptoms of hyperarousal, and avoidance of stimuli associated with the traumatic event. A combination of approaches can be used to treat this, such as group therapy and medication.

Complex PTSD

This is sometimes called a disorder of extreme stress or complicated PTSD, and it is normally something that is experienced by persons who have been exposed to traumatic circumstances over a prolonged time, such as domestic abuse. People with this type of PTSD often also diagnosed with borderline or antisocial personality disorders. They typically exhibit behavioral problems such as aggression, eating disorders, drug and alcohol abuse, and impulsivity. This person might often experience extreme emotions such as intense rage depression and panic and have difficulties with mental functions such as disassociation, amnesia, and fragmented thoughts. Persons with this type of PTSD often take longer to respond to treatment and require a highly structured treatment program to gain results.

Comorbid PTSD

This type of PTSD is normally associated with another major psychiatric disorder such as alcohol and substance abuse, depression, and anxiety disorder. The best method of treatment is to treat both of these disorders at the same time. Typically methods of treatment that work with uncomplicated PTSD work in this circumstance as well.

How to Cope With PTSD Using Your Breath

While it might be difficult to get your life back on track if you have suffered PTSD, it is possible with short-term and long-term treatment options. These treatment options include medications and psychotherapy. While medication might be useful in treating the more extreme emotional and mental symptoms such as depression and emotional outbursts, psychotherapy helps teach the person how to deal with the symptoms. Implementing practical exercises learned here will help restore their self-esteem and self-confidence in dealing with everyday situations.

One of the long-term strategies that you can use, which is safe, natural, and effective is, of course, breathwork. Here are breathing techniques you can employ to help with PTSD symptoms.

Soft Focus Breathing

This breathing technique helps control the fight-or-flight response, which is easily triggered in a person with PTSD. To practice this technique, ensure that you are comfortable and sit cross-legged on a soft mat, chair, or bed. Put your hands on your face with your hands facing upward. Close your eyes and breathe in deeply and slowly through your nose. Allow the air to be guided to your diaphragm. Do this for a count on seven then release the air in a slow exhale through the mouth. Exhale for a count of seven so that you have balanced oxygen intake and carbon dioxide release. As you inhale, mentally project the image of softness to yourself. This can be an image of a cloud, a pillow, or any other object that you associate with softness. This will help direct your mind to a safe space and hence help you relax. This aids in dealing with the emotional and mental turmoil of PTSD symptoms. When you exhale, envision that whatever tension that you carry in your body and mind is being swallowed up by the softness. Do this for 5 minutes two to three times a day or as needed to help you relax. It can be done at bedtime to help you fall asleep faster.

7-11 breathing technique

This technique aids in lowering stress levels and promoting a calm state of mind. It is also as easy as the name suggests. You breathe in for a count of seven and exhale for a count of eleven. Ensure that your inhales go through your diaphragm and that your exhales are pushed out through pursed lips. This technique helps in the controlled release of carbon dioxide and to boost mental function for increased focus and clarity.

Active Breathing

This breathing technique is great for expelling fear, quieting the negative thoughts in your mind with breathwork as well as adjusting your mindset. Start in a standing position with a straight spin and arms at your side. Inhale deeply and slowly for a count of eight. Exhale for a count of eight as well but make a shhh sound when you do this. As you make this sounds, imagine that the thoughts in your head are people and that they respond to this sound by being quiet. The sound is also useful in opening up the diagram, which can close up when fear, anxiety, and stress are being felt. This limits the air volume that is taken into the body and so normal body and mental function.

Calming Breathing

In a standing position with your arms at your side and your spine straight, inhale through your nose for a count of seven. Allow the air to go to your diagram. Exhale through your nose and make an mmm sound as the air leaves your nostrils. Keep your lips closed to build the pressure so that the sound causes a vibration through your head. The vibration stimulates a nerve called the vagus nerve, which is located in the main branch of the parasympathetic nervous system. The vagus nerve happens to be the longest in the body and connects the brain to many important organs. It influences your breathing, digestive function, and more. Therefore, stimulating the vagus nerve allows the over-aroused nervous system to relax so that the PTSD patient can have improved clarity of thought and focus among its many benefits.

Other Meditation Practices for Trauma Therapy

The mind-body technique of meditation can also aid in relieving the symptoms of PTSD. The symptoms of PTSD such as flashbacks, anxiety, anger, mental confusion, and more are a bid the mind makes to ensure the survival of the individual involved. The mind floods the entire system of that human beings with sensations, images, emotions, and perceptions meant to keep that person alive. Therefore, meditation is a great way of refocusing that mental energy into a daily function rather than focusing on survival. Meditation encourages mental calm and self-awareness so that the person can move past the thoughts and feelings in their head to a better understanding of why their mind and body are reacting the way they are. It is only then that this person can employ strategies to help them cope and move past the trauma. Here are a few meditation exercises you can use to cope with the symptoms of PTSD.

Mindful Meditation for PTSD

The unpleasant thoughts and feelings that are associated with PTSD can distract from living in the moment. This takes away a person's joy and fulfillment and diverts it from where it should be, which is in the present and not in the past. Practicing mindful meditation can help get that person back in touch with the present as well as reduce the control that these unpleasant thoughts and feelings have on them. Mindful meditation also reduces stress and anxiety, both of which are conditions that are related to PTSD. The same routine in Chapter 3: Meditation to Reduce Anxiety: A Simple Mindful Meditation Exercise can be used and is just as effective in this instance.

Progressive Muscle Relaxation for PTSD

Our muscles natural tense in preparation for fight-or-flight mode when we are stressed and anxiety as like with PTSD suffering. Actively getting your muscles to relax can help alleviate the PTSD symptoms. To do this, get to a standing position. Ensure that your spine is straight. This technique relies on tensing up various parts of your body, then releasing that tension. Begin by inhaling for a count of eight. Ensure that the breath goes to your diaphragm. Hold the tension in your entire body for the inhale then let it go as you exhale for a count of eight. Exhale through pursed lips. Next, breathe and tense, then relax specific parts of your body. Start with your neck and throat. Next, perform the procedure on your shoulders, hands, and arms. The belly comes next then the leg and feet. Repeat the breathing process on each body area twice. When you exhale, imagine the tenseness melting off you like butter that has been heated. Finally, after you have performed the procedure over your entire body, continue breathing in and out for counts of eight, five more times. Sway from side to side as you do this so that you expel any lingering tension

Bamboo Swaying

This is also a meditative practice that is great for releasing muscle tension.

Standing still with spine straight and your hands on your thighs in front of you, breathe in through your nose and out through pursed lips deeply and slowly. As you breathe, allow your chin to move forward until your upper body is bent enough to create an arch in your back. Pause there and exhale slowly for a count of eight. Allow your head to fall back and bring your tailbone forward slowly. Round your back and slowly return to an upright position. Repeat this three more times then begin to sway like a bamboo plant in a gentle breeze. Do this slowly and gently to dispel any tension that you are carrying. Pay attention to the movement and feeling in your spine.

Grounded Meditation

This practice is useful for expelling negative emotions and energy. It is an imaginary based exercise and starts with the practitioner standing straight with a straight spine and arms at the side. Keep your eyes open but allow them to defocus so that you are not really looking at anything. As you breathe in through your nose and out through pursed lips slowly and deeply, rise onto your toes then let yourself fall back down to your heels. Imagine that the entire weight drops down when your heels touch the floor. Imagine that this has a heavy sound and picture your negative emotions falling away with that weight. Keep repeating that rise and fall slowly as you breathe naturally and rhythmically. Continue this process for 1 minute.

Conclusion

Our breath is the foundation of life. It sets the rhythm of all our existence, from the time we take our first inhale after birth to our last exhale. In our busy routines, filled with responsibilities, we live disconnected from this wonderful tool to calm ourselves and anchor the mind in the present moment. The breath is the absolute constant to which we can always return when needed.

When we start to pay more attention to the breath, a lifelong journey has begun. The beauty of the breath journey is that it has no endpoint, but the benefits are felt in all stages. By being more mindful with our breath, we can enjoy the present moment, ease feelings of anxiety and depression, improve sleeping patterns, and live a more confident and happier life overall.

Deep Breath begins with the foundational work. Finding better posture and fostering nose breathing are the very first steps in this journey and you will be feeling the benefits in your physical and mental wellbeing every step of the way. You can move through the techniques here presented as slow or as fast as it makes sense to you. This is also a journey of trusting yourself and your body to know what is best for you.

With this guide to breathwork, we have reviewed the main breathing techniques taught today, providing easy-to-follow instructions on each breathwork exercise. From easy two minutes stretches you can practice at your office desk, to relaxing breathing techniques you can bring with yourself in stressful situations, to modern community-based lifestyle approaches, there is something for every routine. You can use this as a toolkit to determine which breathing technique will better soothe your anxiety, boost self-esteem, improve energy levels, or help you deal with grief and loss.

This guide is meant to assist you in finding the right path to a better relationship with your breath and not to prescribe the best approach to everyone. You can come back to our guided meditations and step-by-step breathing instructions until you have found the right approach for you, and even later whenever you want some extra grounding in your breath practice.

This is an individual journey. We have just presented some of the tools available. Maybe you will start your days with ten deep belly breaths. Maybe you will resort to Ujjayi breath anytime you need to find the confidence to make hard decisions. Or you may practice breath of fire before decisive moments.

Breathwork should adapt to you, not the other way around. Learning how to breathe mindfully and intently also entails finding a way to integrate breathwork in our routines in a way that feels organic and feasible. Learning how to have better posture is breathwork. Taking five belly breaths while waiting for the bus is breathwork. So is practicing Ujjayi while jogging and listening to music. With time, you will notice that your body organically takes on these lessons and applies them even without the conscious decision to practice mindful breathing.

Whether you decide to incorporate breathwork during workouts, to take a few moments each day to pay attention to your breath, or to create a consistent breath practice, we hope this guide has helped you to breathe more intentionally, and more importantly, breathe deep.